Minor Surgery in Orthodontics

Edited by
Jean-Paul Schatz, DDS
Jean-Pierre Joho, DDS, MS

University of Geneva
School of Dental Medicine
Department of Orthodontics and Pedodontics
Geneva, Switzerland

Quintessence Publishing Co, Inc
Chicago, Berlin, London, São Paulo, Tokyo, and Hong Kong

Library of Congress Cataloging-in-Publication Data

Minor surgery in orthodontics / [edited by] Jean-Paul Schatz, Jean-Pierre Joho.

Includes bibliographical references and index.
ISBN 0-86715-248-6
1. Mouth—Surgery. 2. Teeth—Abnormalities—Surgery. 3. Orthodontics, Corrective. I. Schatz,
Jean-Paul. II. Joho, Jean-Pierre.
[DNLM: 1. Orthodontics—methods. 2. Surgery, Oral—methods. WU400 M666]
RK529.M56 1992
617.6'43059-dc20
DNLM/DLC
for Library of Congress

92-21163
CIP

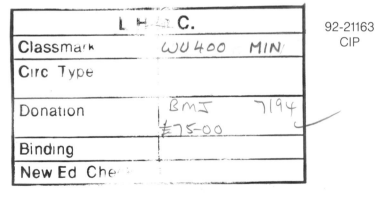
© 1992 by Quintessence Publishing Co., Inc., Chicago, Illinois.
All rights reserved.

Lithography: Industrie- und Presseklischee, Berlin
Typesetting, printing and binding: Bartels & Wernitz, Munich

Printed in Germany

ISBN 0-86715-248-6

Contents

Contributors

Jan van Aken
Professor
Department of Oral and Maxillofacial
Radiology
University of Utrecht
Utrecht, Netherlands

Jean-Pierre Joho
Professor
Department of Orthodontics and
Pedodontics
School of Dental Medicine, University of
Geneva
Geneva, Switzerland

Donald R. Joondeph
Professor
Department of Orthodontics
University of Washington
Seattle, Washington, USA

Daniel M. Laskin
Professor
Department of Oral and Maxillofacial
Surgery
Medical College of Virginia
Richmond, Virginia, USA

Barbro Malmgren
Associate Professor
Eastmaninstitutet Stockholm
Dalagatan 11
S-11324 Stockholm

Olle Malmgren
Associate Professor
Eastmaninstitutet Stockholm
Dalagatan 11
S-11324 Stockholm

Sabine C. Maréchaux
Senior Lecturer
Department of Orthodontics and
Pedodontics
Dental School of Medicine, University of
Geneva
Geneva, Switzerland

Robert M. Ricketts
Director
American Institute for Bioprogressive
Education
Scottsdale, Arizona, USA

Jean-Paul Schatz
Senior Lecturer
Department of Orthodontics and
Pedodontics
School of Dental Medicine, University of
Geneva
Geneva, Switzerland

Robert L. Vanarsdall
Professor
Department of Orthodontics
School of Dental Medicine, University of
Pennsylvania
Philadelphia, Pennsylvania, USA

Foreword

The theme of this timely volume is "the team." It is clear now that no specialists in dentistry can be all things to all patients. The era has passed when the orthodontic specialist was the sole provider of orthodontic treatment. No longer can he be an "island" unto himself. The ramifications of varying ideologies and the multiplicity of therapeutic approaches make it imperative that we have a broad understanding of potential therapeutic approaches that can optimize service to our patients. In its nine chapters, this book admirably addresses that theme to prepare the clinician for orthodontics of today and tomorrow.

Chapter 1 on "Orthodontics and Related Dental Pathology" incisively addresses the issue of environmental versus hereditary factors in the etiology of malocclusion. If we are to render better service, then we have to recognize departures from the normal early and intercept them. This chapter better qualifies the clinician to do just that. The illustrations and examples are of top quality, giving maximum impact and portent in the 18 pages allotted. Prevention and interception makes ultimate therapy easy and, as the authors comment, "Integrating the different factors evoked allows the inception of a reasonable orthodontic treatment plan, often associating relative dental fields to solve these minor dental abnormalities."

"Knowledge is power", and Chapter 2 shows how radiologic assessment of problems that arise in developing dentition is essential. Here again, excellent illustrations and advice as to how to obtain the best possible image quality allow the clinician to maximize the information that is available. The teamwork theme is again emphasized in this important contribution to the book.

Chapter 3, in a way, is a continuation of the theme developed in Chapter 1. It discusses congenital absence of permanent teeth and the orthodontic treatment for this condition. Discretionary diagnostic decisions must be made, in most cases the earlier the better. Long-term records are used to show the results of proper treatment planning. A number of secondary considerations in treatment planning are discussed, i e, canine substitution for the lateral incisor, maxillary lip plank, the need for occlusal equilibration with space closure, etc. Three case reports elucidate the many factors involved in the management of congenital absence problems.

Chapter 4 emphasizes the intraoperative principles of oral surgery and points out the importance of preoperative preparation of the patient and proper postoperative care. Particularly with the great increase in orthognathic surgery being done, such teamwork between the oral surgeon and orthodontist is imperative. The medical background is important and often determines the type of anesthesia,

7

the therapeutic approach, etc. Recent emphasis on sterilization because of the spread of AIDS and hepatitis viruses makes the section on asepsis in this chapter particularly valuable. The management of soft and hard tissues is covered. As the author states, "Understanding the basic principles of surgery also helps in explaining failures when they occur."

Chapter 5, "Anatomy and Morphology of the Periodontium" and Chapter 6, "Orthodontic/Periodontal Considerations for Minor Periodontal Surgery," are perfect examples of the great need for teamwork today. The author, with dual specialty training in orthodontics and periodontics, is one of the world's leaders in this field. These chapters are a "must" for any orthodontist practicing today. Many important anatomic and physiologic considerations are addressed, helping the clinician better control and maintain optimal environmental conditions during tooth movement.

Chapter 7 on "The Dilemma of the Third Molar" discusses the divergent views concerning what to do with third molar teeth and when to do it. According to the author, the controversy may have been caused by lack of criteria for judgment and insufficient knowledge of the method of eruption, the process of growth and space creation, performance of third molars in functional occlusion, conditions causing crowding, and short- and long-term consequences of impaction or erupted complications. The information presented is provocative and will stimulate the reader to pursue the subject further.

Chapter 8 on "Orthodontic Management of Traumatized Teeth" addresses the important questions of pulp vitality, periodontal implications, and technical concerns.

Chapter 9 presents two excellent case reports illustrating the proper approach to these problems. Both chapters 8 and 9 have superb illustrations and excellent bibliographies that will allow further study, and are at the cutting edge of orthodontic surgical teamwork.

Certainly it is a privilege to write a foreword for this fine volume. I know of no book in the literature that has put together this amount of information more succinctly and up to date in 179 pages. It is a literary gem that will undoubtedly be continued with future editions.

T. M. Graber

Chapter 1

Orthodontics and Related Dental Pathology

Sabine C. Maréchaux / Jean-Paul Schatz / Jean-Pierre Joho

Because knowledge of the normal and abnormal development of the denture is a prerequisite for any orthodontic treatment planning, the depiction of various minor pathologies may also be of significance.[1] Any deviation from the normal is considered to be an anomaly and can be hereditary, congenital or due to environmental factors. It may affect the developing dentition in changes of number, shape, color, and structure of teeth; eruption and exfoliation; and position. Environmental influences include radiation exposure, medication, or maternal avitaminoses during pregnancy, and external injurious factors during tooth formation, such as trauma and infections.

Anomalies of number

Hyperodontia and hypodontia are obviously related to other specific clinical situations, including dentoalveolar problems such as dental crowding or diastemata. They usually affect the distal tooth of each kind (ie, second premolar, third molar, etc), with the exception of the mandibular anterior area, where the central incisors are missing more often than the lateral incisors.

Hyperodontia is a rare condition in primary dentition; missing or retained primary teeth are more common and may be followed by missing permanent teeth.

Aplasia of one or more teeth is a frequent reason orthodontic consultation is made and has far-reaching effects on orthodontic treatments.

Hyperodontia

If not related to genetic factors or syndromes, hyperodontia can be explained by cellular hyperactivity or tissue duplication. Present primarily in permanent dentition, its frequency varying with its location, a supernumerary tooth is a real orthodontic concern if its impaction impedes the normal eruption of a tooth or induces a malocclusion.

The prevalence of supernumerary teeth in the primary dentition varies from 0.3 % to 1.8 % (Fig. 1-1), is usually restricted to the incisor region and does not necessarily repeat itself in the permanent dentition. The prevalence of supernumerary teeth in the permanent dentition varies from 2 % to 3 %.[2] They are located mainly in the maxillary incisor region, with a lower percentage in the premolar area, and there appears to be a higher incidence in boys than in girls.

9

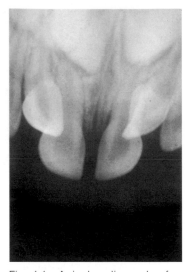

Fig. 1-1 Apical radiograph of a 3-year-old girl with two maxillary primary supernumerary lateral incisors.

The presence of multiple supernumerary and retained primary teeth, as seen in Fig. 1-3, is typical of cleidocranial dysostosis. The extraction of the retained primary teeth does not necessarily induce the eruption of the permanent teeth, and therefore the primary dentition should be restored and maintained for as long as possible.

Hypodontia

Hypodontia is more frequent in permanent than in primary dentition and is often associated with more severe syndromes (CLP, ectodermal dysplasia) (Fig. 1-4). Its frequency seems to be increasing and indicates a trend toward a reduction of available maxillary space for the human dentition.[3] Hypodontia in the primary dentition is present in less than 1% of the studies recorded in the literature (Fig. 1-5).

Anodontia and oligodontia, total or almost complete absence of teeth, are often associated with ectodermal dysplasia.[4,5] Figure 1-5 shows a frontal view of a 4-year-old boy with congenitally missing maxillary primary lateral incisors and mandibular primary incisors. In addition, the maxillary primary central incisors are peg shaped.

In the permanent dentition, the most common supernumerary tooth, and the most atypical in morphology, is the mesiodens (Fig.1-2a and b). Mesiodentes are frequently associated with an abnormal or retained position of one or both central incisors.

Figs. 1-2a and b   Clinical and radiologic views of a maxillary right mesiodens in a 7-year-old boy.

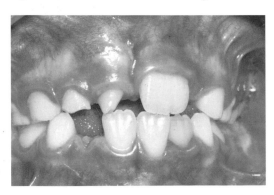
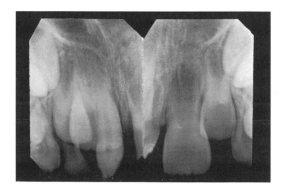

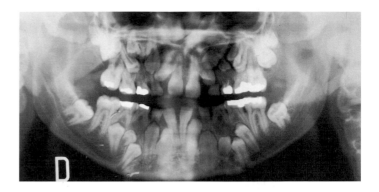

Fig. 1-3 Panoramic radiograph of a patient with cleidocranial dysostosis: none of the permanent lateral incisors, canines, or premolars have erupted. There are supernumerary permanent premolars in both the maxilla and mandible.

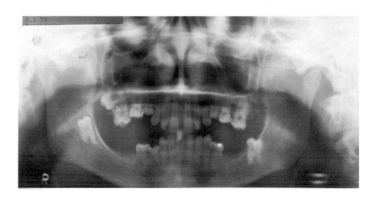

Fig. 1-4 Panoramic radiograph of a 16-year-old girl with oligodontia, ankylosed primary teeth, and impacted permanent teeth, without obvious related syndrome.

Fig. 1-5 A 4-year-old boy with aplasia of mandibular primary incisors and maxillary primary lateral incisors; in addition, the maxillary primary central incisors are peg shaped.

Fig. 1-6 Single central maxillary primary incisor. The central incisor is a central tooth, ie, the mesial and distal sides are symmetric.

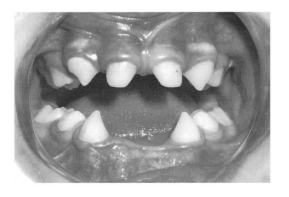

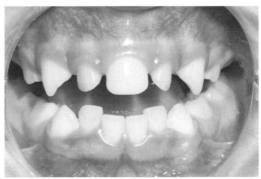

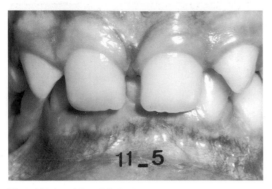
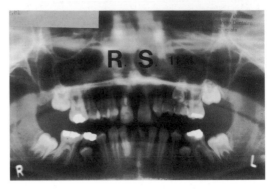

Figs. 1-7a and b   Clinical and radiologic views showing missing maxillary permanent lateral incisors and mandibular permanent central incisors.

Other physical aspects of ectodermal dysplasia are fine, scanty hair; partial or complete absence of sweat glands with resultant fine, smooth and dry skin; protuberant lips; and a depressed bridge of the nose.

Cases of cleft lip and palate also exhibit a higher frequency of congenitally missing permanent teeth, especially in the maxillary permanent lateral incisor area.

An unusual kind of hypodontia is seen in Fig. 1-6. This 4-year-old boy has a single maxillary primary central incisor. The condition is extremely rare and sometimes attributed to a lack of growth hormone.[6,7] The maxillary primary incisor is a central tooth, ie, the mesial and distal sides are identical. Of all the hypodontias, the maxillary central incisor is the tooth that is missing the least frequently, accounting for only 0.66%. The highest percentage of hypodontia, with the exception of third molar, is attributed to mandibular permanent second premolars (47.3%), followed by the maxillary permanent second premolar (25.3%). The next most commonly congenitally missing permanent tooth is the maxillary lateral incisor, with an incidence of 12.3%.

Because the stages of mineralization for maxillary lateral incisors are remarkably stable, aplasia of these teeth can be diagnosed as early as age 4. Even the aplasia of second premolars, which can develop as late as age 12, could also be ruled out early with a high degree of fiability.

Hypodontia often requires orthodontic and restorative treatments, as seen in the case of an 11-year-old girl with congenitally missing maxillary permanent lateral incisors and mandibular permanent central incisors (Figs. 1-7a and b). The latter account for only 2.2% of the anodontias.

Four years later, at the end of the orthodontic treatment, the maxillary permanent canines were restored with composite resin to the anatomical morphology of lateral incisors (Fig. 1-8). The spaces were closed in the mandibular arch, with permanent lateral incisors and canines aligned as an incisal unit.

Anomalies of shape

Morphologic deviations are mostly genetically dictated and concern to somewhat

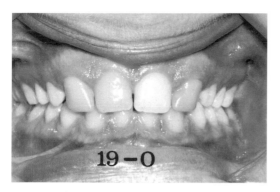

Fig. 1-8 At the end of orthodontic treatment, the spaces of the missing mandibular incisors have been closed and the maxillary permanent canines have been restored to lateral incisors.

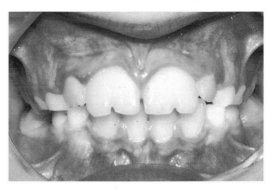

Fig. 1-9 Gemination of maxillary permanent central incisors, inducing esthetic, orthodontic, and periodontal problems.

the same extent both primary and permanent dentition. With the exception of fusion of temporary teeth which often prefigurate hypodontia in permanent dentition, those anomalies in morphology do not bear any prognostic value on morphology in late permanent dentition. They can, though, hinder the development of normal occlusion, especially by creating discrepancies in tooth size. It seems that even the cases showing crowding in permanent dentition have teeth with an average larger size, reflecting probably the lack of genetic relationship between the size of the maxilla and that of the teeth.

As with anomalies of number, there can be modifications in the morphology of the teeth, which originate in the proliferation stage of tooth development. These can be additional canines or roots, especially on molars and premolars; fusion, defined as an incomplete attempt of two tooth buds to fuse into one; or gemination, which is the incomplete attempt of a tooth bud to divide (Fig. 1-9).

The etiology of fusion has been described as a physical pressure leading to the subsequent uniting of teeth. Its fre-

quency appears to be 0.5 % in the primary dentition and 0.1 % in the permanent dentition.[8,9] There is no sex difference, and the malformation is restricted to the canine-incisor region. In the primary dentition, Ravn[2] quotes more fusion in the mandible and more gemination in the maxilla. The malformation may be bilateral but does not necessarily repeat itself in the permanent dentition.

Shape anomalies include many other disorders, such as dilaceration, Hutchinson's incisors, and Mulberry molars caused by congenital syphilis; peg laterals; dens-in-dente; taurodontism; macrodontia and microdontia; hypoplastic defects; and malformation resulting from trauma, exanthematous diseases, and genetic syndromes.

While microdontia is relatively common when a single tooth is involved (Figs. 1-10 and 1-11), usually the maxillary permanent lateral incisor or third molar, true generalized microdontia is rare except in some cases of pituitary dwarfism.[10] Figures 1-12 and 1-13 show the case of a 20-year-old female with true generalized microdontia, anodontia of the mandibular permanent

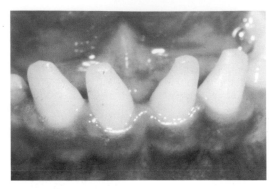

Fig. 1-10 Microdontia of mandibular permanent incisors.

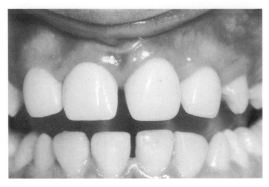

Fig. 1-11 Frontal view of the same patient following orthodontic treatment and restoration of the mandibular and maxillary permanent incisors.

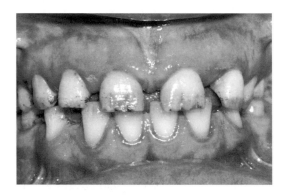

Fig. 1-12 A 20-year-old girl with true generalized microdontia.

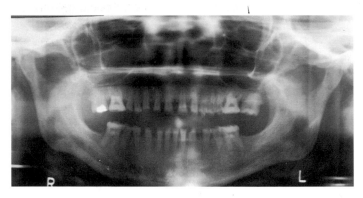

Fig. 1-13 Panoramic radiograph shows the aplasia of the mandibular permanent second molars and of all third molars, in addition to the microdontia.

second and third molars, and enamel hypoplasia. This patient's generalized microdontia may be attributed to a congenital anemia, which also led to dwarfism and other physical malformations.

Anomalies of color and structure

Even slight perturbations of mineral concentration in the blood flow can affect the permanent dentition, despite the regulating factors probably acting on a local level. These temporary or long-term problems usually result in spots, colorations, cracks, etc, which indicate the stage of mineralization where problems occurred.

A severe trauma in primary dentition can also be followed by various pathologies in permanent dentition or, in some circumstances, prevent root formation by a break-up in the mineralization process.

Changes in color can be either extrinsic or intrinsic.[11,12] Extrinsic stains, usually deposits, can be removed by a thorough prophylaxis. Intrinsic stains have various etiologic factors, all of which interfered in the histodifferentiation stage of tooth development and are expressed by different discolorations:
1. Yellow — tetracycline, premature birth, amelogenesis imperfecta
2. Brown — tetracycline, amelogenesis and dentinogenesis imperfecta, premature birth, cystic fibrosis, and porphyria
3. Blue to green — erythroblastosis fetalis
4. White — fluorosis, snow-capped teeth, idiopathic opacities, amelogenesis imperfecta
5. Red to brown — porphyria

6. Gray to brown — dentinogenesis imperfecta, traumatic injuries, systemic diseases

Congenital dentinogenesis imperfecta is also known as hereditary opalescent dentin and occurs when the mesodermal part of the odontogenic apparatus is disturbed, leading to defective dentin deposits. Because of an abnormal dentino-enamel junction, the enamel is lost and the dentin undergoes attrition, with partial or total pulpal obliteration. In addition there is a loss of vertical dimension, as can be seen in the posterior areas (Figs. 1-14 and 1-15). Treatment modalities aim at restoring the vertical dimension by either full crown rehabilitation or overdentures.

Dentinogenesis imperfecta[13] may be associated with osteogenesis imperfecta, in which there is hardly any development of the long bony structures and a high risk of fractures results. These children usually do not outlive puberty.

Amelogenesis imperfecta[13] (Fig. 1-16), a systemic disease characterized by defective ameloblasts, may be due to an acute sensitivity to an unidentified factor and is sometimes linked to other ectodermal defects. Its occurrence has been reported to be 1:14,000 to 1:16,000.

Clinical features of the disease are:
1. Varying number of teeth involved, affecting the primary and/or the permanent dentition
2. A deficiency in enamel thickness, with normal to yellow discoloration; teeth are small with no interproximal contact points
3. Attrition and resultant loss of vertical dimension, the enamel separating from the underlying dentin

Patients are usually caries-free, because the anatomic forms of the teeth contribute

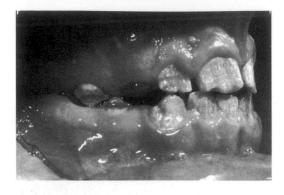

Fig. 1-14 An 11-year-old girl with dentinogenesis imperfecta and associated loss of vertical dimension.

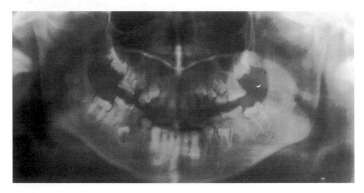

Fig. 1-15 Panoramic radiograph shows the typical dentin malformations.

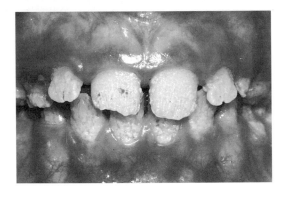

Fig. 1-16 A 9-year-old girl with amelogenesis imperfecta.

to self-cleansing. In some cases, however, brushing is painful, resulting in poor hygiene and gingivitis. Painful mastication may also lead to weight loss. A radiographic view of the same patient (Fig. 1-17) shows the defective enamel formation on all the permanent teeth and on the remaining primary teeth, while dentin and root formation is normal.

Dentinal dysplasia and shell teeth are two other types of extremely rare anomalies of structure. Dentinal dysplasia, ac-

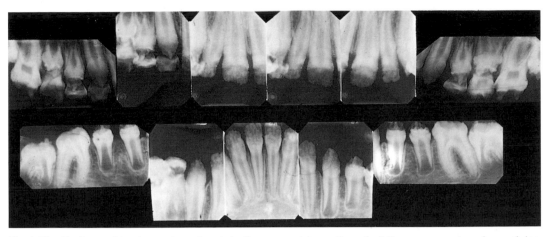

Fig. 1-17   Radiographic views show the defective enamel formation of all the permanent and remaining primary teeth.

cording to Shafer et al,[14] is a disturbance of dentin formation characterized by normal enamel, highly atypical dentin with pulpal obliteration, defective root formation, and a tendency for periapical pathology. It appears to be a hereditary disease affecting both the primary and permanent dentition. Pulp cavities and root canals are obliterated much earlier than in dentinogenesis imperfecta, excluding proper endodontic therapy. Because of the anatomic restrictions and the periapical involvement, the usual outcome is premature exfoliation of the teeth.[15]

Shell teeth is a form of dental dysplasia in which the enamel appears normal, while the dentin is extremely thin and the pulp cavities enormous. These teeth also have short roots, but the syndrome does not appear to be hereditary.

Anomalies of eruption and exfoliation

A thorough knowledge of the mechanism and sequence of eruption and of the different stages of mineralization is mandatory for a sound and proper timing of any orthodontic treatment planning, especially for interceptive cases and those involving serial extractions. A radiologic screening should allow localization of various pathologies (supernumerary, aplasias, etc) and permit distinction between late eruption and impactions.

Anomalies of eruption

The perturbations of eruption, if severe, are usually related to some general illnesses or syndromes and can be classified as premature or retarded eruption.

A premature eruption is rather rare[16] and due mainly to hormonal disturbances, such as hyperthyroidism. It can also be due to hypophosphatasia,[17] where a decreased alkaline phosphatase activity with resultant vitamin D deficiency leads to a perturbed cementogenesis of the primary teeth. There is no functional periodontal attachment, with the resultant loosening of the teeth.

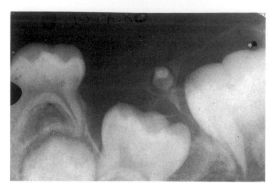

Fig. 1-18   Apical radiograph of an ankylosed mandibular primary left second molar of a 5-year-old girl, associated to a supernumerary tooth.

Retarded eruption can be due to local factors,[18] such as a fibrous gingiva, supernumerary and impacted teeth, ankylosis, crowding, or ectopic eruption. To the same extent, hormonal disturbances such as hypothyroidism or hypoparathyroidism, Down's syndrome, nutritional disturbances such as vitamin A and D deficiency (rickets), or infectious disorders, such as congenital syphilis, may be causative factors.

Ankylosis

Ankylosis in primary and secondary dentition is the result of local perturbations of mostly unknown origin and affect the evolution of permanent dentition as well as the alveolar growth processes.[19]

The etiology of tooth ankylosis has been attributed to a congenital gap in the periodontal membrane of genetic or localized trauma origin, or to a locally disturbed arrhythmic metabolism. While ankylosis is located mainly in the primary molar area during the mixed dentition stage,[20] with an incidence of 1.9% to 14.3%, permanent molars may also be affected. The ratio of primary teeth to permanent teeth is 10:1, with a predilection for mandibular arch location.

Because ankylosis usually concerns the primary molars, it necessitates extraction only if the observed infraocclusion can lead to impaction or to excessive tipping of adjacent teeth (Fig. 1-18).[21-23]

In cases of permanent molar ankylosis, a surgical mobilization associated with an orthodontic extrusion can sometimes be successful. Most of the time, however, re-ankylosis is the rule and extraction the only therapeutic choice. In those cases, as well as in those of missing teeth, orthodontic closure mechanisms have been claimed as an ideal solution in selected clinical situations.

Anomalies of exfoliation

Premature exfoliation of the primary teeth can be due to radiation exposure, especially following radiation therapy, leukemia, juvenile periodontitis, odonto-hypophosphatasia, vitamin D—resistant rickets, Hand-Schüller-Christian disease, and Letterer-Siwe disease.

Retarded exfoliation of the primary dentition is associated mainly with cleidocranial dysostosis and Down's syndrome, whereas localized retarded exfoliation can be due to ankylosis or impaction.

Both premature or retarded exfoliation of primary teeth can modify the clinical eruption sequence of permanent dentition and consequently lead to various malocclusion.[24]

Anomalies of position

Anomalies of position may be due to impaction, ankylosis, undermining resorption, transposition, deleterious oral habits, gingival hyperplasia, and, most commonly, a lack of space for the erupting permanent dentition. They represent the major source of orthodontic consultation and are related to the development of the denture, in as much as any pathology (ankylosis, supernumerary teeth, cysts, etc) can directly modify the erupting pathway of a tooth. Among them, impactions, ectopic eruptions and transpositions are the most common. Ectopic eruption usually involves the maxillary canines, which may erupt mesial to the lateral incisors or distal to the first premolars (ie, transposition).

Impacted teeth are prevented from eruption by some physical barrier, usually by adjacent teeth (ie, mandibular second premolars) or by a supernumerary tooth.[25] An abnormal direction of eruption, the rotation of a tooth bud or a generalized lack of space available for eruption can also lead to permanent inclusion. Some pathologic entities, tumors or cysts, can also affect the normal course of eruption in permanent dentition, most often leading to definitive impactions.

The most frequently impacted teeth are third molars and maxillary canines, followed by premolars and supernumerary teeth. In a study of 3,874 routine full-mouth radiographs, the incidence of impacted maxillary third molars was 22 %, and that of mandibular third molars was 18 %. Thilander and Jacobsson,[26] and Ericson and Kurol,[27] reported a prevalence of approximately 2 % of impacted maxillary canines, most of them in palatal position. While the treatment of choice for impacted third molars is surgical removal, impacted maxillary canines can be transplanted or surgically exposed and brought into occlusal alignment by orthodontic treatment.[28, 29]

In the anterior area, maxillary central or lateral incisors can be considered impacted if not erupted one year after full eruption of their contralaterals. Apart from an ectopic position of the tooth bud, the presence of supernumerary teeth, cysts, fibrous tissues subsequent to a trauma and crowding are the most frequent causes of impaction (Figs. 1-19a to c).

A careful full-mouth radiologic survey is a major step for planning the orthodontic treatment of those cases: the surgical extraction of a supernumerary tooth, once space reopening and midline shift corrections have been completed, offers good chances of spontaneous correction, though an orthodontic disimpaction with fixed or removable appliances is usually associated to avoid a surgical reentry.

Undermining resorption is characteristic of a maxillary permanent first molar blocked beneath the distal enamel cervical ridge of the maxillary primary second molar because of improper guidance during its eruption.[30, 31] The undermining resorption may be the cause of premature exfoliation of the primary second molar and subsequent space loss: an observation period of 4 to 6 months is recommended because spontaneous correction is observed in half of the cases.

On the contrary, if there is no associated orthodontic problem requiring extractions, a short treatment is undertaken to upright the concerned molar and reopen the space for the second premolar's eruption. Rinderer[32] quoted an incidence of 6 % of undermining resorption of primary second molars, mostly in the maxilla, rising to 25 %

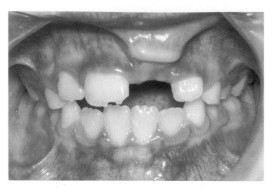

Fig. 1-19a   Impaction of the left maxillary central incisor following trauma in the primary dentition.

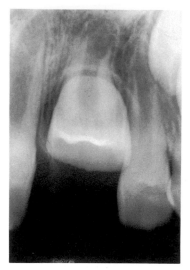

Fig.   1-19b Apical   radiograph showing horizontal impaction of tooth 21.

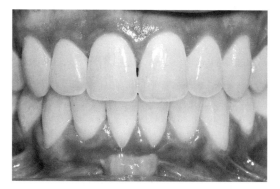

Fig. 1-19c   Clinical view at the end of orthodontic treatment.

in cleft lip and palate cases. Undermining resorption may also be observed in cases of erupting permanent molars, especially third molars.

Summary

The various above-mentioned pathologic entities point out the delicate equilibrium needed to achieve a stable and functional dentition that even a minor perturbation can affect. Integrating the different factors evoked allow the inception of a reasonable orthodontic treatment plan, often associating related dental fields to solve these minor dental abnormalities.

References

1. Lundström A. Malocclusion of the teeth: classification, prevalence, aetiology and treatment need. In: Thilander and Rönning (eds): *Introduction to Orthodontics*. Stockholm: Tandläkarförlaget; 1985.

2. Ravn J J. Aplasia, supernumerary teeth and fused teeth in the primary dentition: An epidemiologic study. *Scand J Dent Res* 1971; 79:1–6.

3. Proffit W R. *Contemporary Orthodontics*. St Louis: C. V. Mosby Company; 1986.

4. Silverman E, Ackerman J L. Oligodontia. A study of its prevalence and variation in 4032 children. *J Dent Child* 1979; 46:470–477.

5. Suarez B K, Spence M A. The genetics of hypodontia. *J Dent Res* 1974; 53:781–785.

6. Rappaport E B, Ulstrom R A, Gorlin R J et al. Solitary maxillary central incisor and short stature. *J Pediatr* 1977; 91:924–928.

7. Santoro F P, Wesley R K. Clinical evaluation of two patients with a single maxillary contral incisor. *J Dent Child* 1983; 50:379–381.

8. Maréchaux S C. The treatment of fusion of a maxillary central incisor and a supernumerary, Report of a case. *J Dent Child* 1984; 51:196–199.

9. Croll T P, Jackson R N, Chen E. Fusion and gemination in one dental arch, Report of a case. *J Dent Child* 1981; 48:297–299.

10. Joho J P, Maréchaux S C. Microdontia, A specific tooth anomaly, Report of a case. *J Dent Child* 1979; 46:483–486.

11. Hayes P A, Full C, Pinkham J. The etiology and treatment of intrinsic discoloration. *J Can Dent Assoc* 1986; 52:217–220.

12. Giunta J L, Tsamtsouris A. Stains and discolorations of teeth: Review and case report. *J Pedod* 1978; 2:175–182.

13. Joho J P, Maréchaux S C. Amelogenesis imperfecta, Treatment of a case. *J Dent Child* 1980; 47:266–268.

14. Shafer W G, Hine M K, Levy B M. *A Textbook of Oral Pathology,* Philadelphia and London: W. B. Saunders Company; 1963.

15. Logan J, Becks H, Silverman S, Pindborg J J. Dentinal Dysplasia. *Oral Surg Oral Med Oral Pathol* 1962; 15:317–333.

16. Bjuggren G. Premature eruption in the primary dentition: A clinical and radiological study. *Swed Dent J* 1973; 66:343–353.

17. Beumer J, Silverman S, Eisenberg E. Childhood hypophosphatasia and the premature loss of teeth. *Oral Surg Oral Med Oral Pathol* 1973; 35:631–640.

18. Johnsen D C. Prevalence of delayed emergence of permanent teeth as a result of local factors. *J Am Dent Assoc* 1977; 94:100–106.

19. Biedermann W. Etiology and treatment of tooth ankylosis. *Am J Orthod* 1962; 48:670–684.

20. Kurol J. Infraocclusion of primary molars. *Swed Dent J* 1984; Suppl 21.

21. Steigmann S, Koyoumdjisky-Kaye F, Matrai Y. Relationship of submerged deciduous molars to root resorption and development of permanent successors. *J Dent Res* 1974; 53:88–93.

22. Messer L B, Cline J T. Ankylosed primary molars: results and treatment recommendations from an eight-year longitudinal study. *Pediatr Dent* 1980; 2:37–47.

23. Fanning E A. Effect of extraction of deciduous molars on formation and eruption of their successors. *Angle Orthod* 1962; 32:44–55.

24. Kerr W J S. The effect of the premature loss of deciduous canines and molars on the eruption of their successors. *Europ J Orthod* 1980; 2:123–128.

25. Thilander B, Thilander H. Impacted premolars. *Trans Eur Orthod Soc* 1976; 167–175.

26. Thilander B, Jacobsson S O. Local factors in impaction of maxillary canines. *Acta Odont Scand* 1968; 26:145–168.

27. Ericson S L, Kurol J. Early extraction of palatally erupting maxillary canines by extraction of the primary canines. *Europ J Orthod* 1988; 10:283–295.

28. Schatz J P, Joho J P. Aspects cliniques et théoriques des réimplantations dentaires. *Med & Hyg* 1986; 44:1418–1421.

29. Joho J P, Schatz J P. Autotransplantation et planification orthodontique. *Rev Mens Suisse Odontostomatol* 1990; 100:174–184.

30. Pulver F. The etiology and prevalence of ectopic eruption of the maxillary first permanent molar. *J Dent Child* 1968; 35:138–146.

31. Bjerklin K, Kurol J. Ectopic eruption of the maxillary first permanent molar: Etiologic factors. *Am J Orthod* 1983; 84:147–155.

32. Rinderer L A. Zur unterminierenden Resorption der zweiten Milchmolaren beim Durchbruch der 6-Jahr-Molaren. *Schweiz Mschr Zahnmed* 1984; 94:471–497.

Chapter 2

Radiologic Assessment for Minor Surgery in Orthodontics

Jan van Aken

When a radiograph is made, the image of the object on the film is produced by a simple way of projection. The projecting rays all start at the focal spot of the x-ray machine and follow straight lines, irrespective of the kind of material penetrated. The projection is therefore governed by straight lines that start at one point, pass through the patient, and reach the film.

The different shades of gray in the radiographic image are produced by differences between the attenuation of the various rays caused by the nonhomogeneous composition of the object penetrated.

Differences in attenuation of the x-ray beam by an object are the result of differences in the atomic composition, the concentration of the different kind of atoms present, and the thickness of the material. When translated into clinical terms, it means that six different kinds of materials can be distinguished on the radiographic film because they attenuate the radiation differently. They are, in order of attenuation: air, soft tissue, bone and dentin, and enamel. To this list must be added the dental materials used in the patient's mouth. They differ in composition, and as a result, large differences in the attenuation of the radiation occur. The image of the materials can

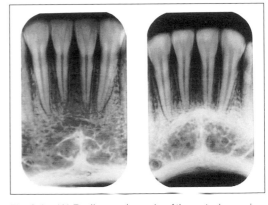

Fig. 2-1 (A) Radiograph made of the anterior region of a mandible using a small vertical angulation of the x-ray beam. (B) Radiograph made of the same area but using a larger vertical angulation of the x-ray beam. On this image the superior slope of the mental ridge is visible.

therefore vary between a very low and a high density (blackening).

In addition to the composition of the tissues, the distance that the rays have to travel through these tissues is important. This factor is determined by the anatomic structure of the patient and the direction of the rays when passing through the patient. The direction of the rays in relation to the patient is the main factor that determines the kind of image that is obtained and the

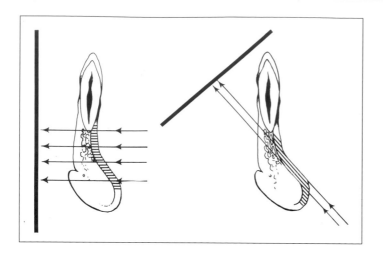

Figs. 2-2a and b   The effect of the direction of the x-ray beam relative to the object on the image obtained. In this example the vertical angulation is changed. (For the images obtained see Fig. 2-1.)

aspects of the structure of the patient that are visualized. Fig. 2-1 shows two images of the same dry specimen of a mandible. The direction of the radiation in relation to the object when the exposures were made was different. The explanation for the differences between the two images is given in Figs. 2-2a and b. It shows that the image obtained depends on the shape of the object and the distance the rays have to travel through the bone. In fact, the image shows a projection of two dimensions of the three-dimensional object on the film, whereas the missing third dimension that influences the attenuation of the beam is registered by the blackening of the film. This blackening in the image is determined by the total attenuation of each ray and does not give information on how this attenuation is distributed along the track of a ray.

Because the aim of the interpretation of the image is to obtain information on the structure of the patient, further information is required to supplement the third dimension.

This missing information can be added

in different ways. Generally the observer supplements the third dimension by making use of (1) his knowledge of the anatomy visualized; (2) knowledge of the direction of the x-ray beam used in the investigation; (3) his experience obtained by the interpretation of images of different patients, which acquaints him with the normal variability in the anatomy; (4) literature dealing with the interpretation of images; (5) his knowledge of the effect of pathologic processes on the structures imaged; and (6) a study of anatomic specimens with or without pathologic conditions in order to find the explanation for aspects in the image he could not understand.

In panoramic tomograms the evaluation of the third dimension is limited to the layer of the object that is visualized (see *Panoramic Tomography*).

Although the practice of this procedure leads in many cases to the desired diagnostic conclusions, it will fail when the diagnostic task involves the determination of the position of isolated objects. This is of special importance in orthodontics when

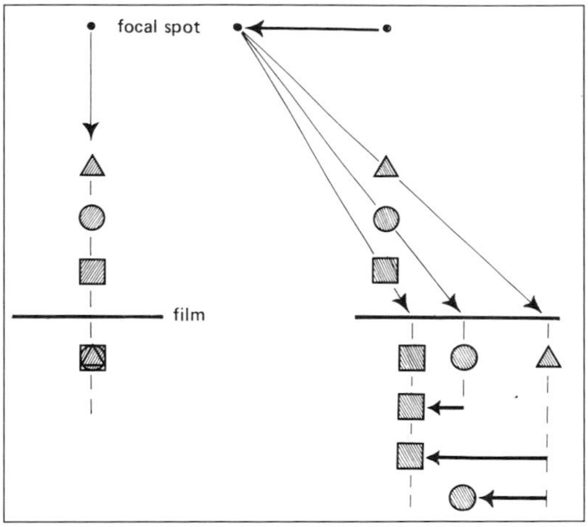

Fig. 2-3 The influence of the position of the focal spot on the relative position of the images of objects that are at different distances from the focal spot. The image of an object, which is closer to the film than a reference object, moves in relation to the image of the reference object in the same direction as the focal spot was moved between the two exposures.

impacted teeth or impacted supernumerary teeth are present. There are five ways to determine the position of these objects.

1. Using two images made at right angles to each other. These two images permit the localization of an object by determining its position in the two images relative to other structures. In principle, the orthogonal x, y, and z space coordinates are read from the films.

2. Using two images made with the x-ray source at two different positions. The location of the object can be found by applying a simple rule. This rule is based on the effect of the movement of the x-ray source between the two exposures on the displacement of the image of the object in relation to a known object or structure that can be observed when the two images are compared. Figure 2-3 explains this relation and makes clear that if the image of the object moves in relation to the known object, in the same direction as the x-ray source between the exposures, it lies behind (lingual to) the known object.

As an aid to memory, this may be called the AXIAL rule (As X-ray Is At Lingual). Figures 2-4a and b show two radiographs that can be used to exercise the application of this rule.

3. Using two images made with the x-ray source at two different positions that correspond approximately with the distance between the eyes of an observer. The two images can be used to produce a stereoscopic view of the patient. Viewing of the stereo-radiographs is possible with a stereoscope. It is also possible to achieve a stereoscopic view without the help of an apparatus by looking at the two images and forcing each eye to look at a different image. It requires exercise to learn to direct the eyes in an abnormal direction, but when this technique is mastered it is rather convenient because it does not require the use of a stereoscope. The correct way of viewing is obtained by taking the following steps (Fig. 2-5). Position the films on the viewbox. Put the tip of a pencil at A (see illustration). The correct position can be checked by looking with one eye at a time. The tip should coincide for each eye with

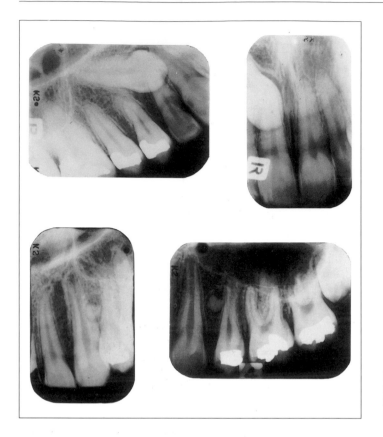

Figs. 2-4a and b Two pairs of radiographs that can be used to determine the relative position of an unerupted tooth.

Fig. 2-5 A method of obtaining a stereoscopic effect. Refer to text for a detailed explanation of this method. Note: the film taken from the "right eye position" is on the left side of the observer. The film taken from the "left eye position" is on the right side of the observer.

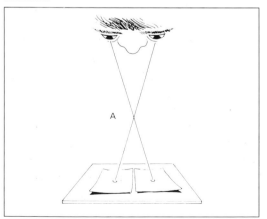

the same structure, which is preferably located at the middle of the film. Look with both eyes at A. After a short time the two images merge into one stereoscopic view. Fig. 2-6a and b show two pairs of images that can be used to exercise this technique.

4. Using a cinematographic recording of a moving or rotating patient in the x-ray beam. With the help of an image intensifier, the projection of such a film makes a strong three-dimensional impression of the object. A disadvantage of this technique is the rather complicated set-up required to make the film. The possibilities of this technique are therefore limited.

5. Using tomography. This technique also requires complicated equipment.

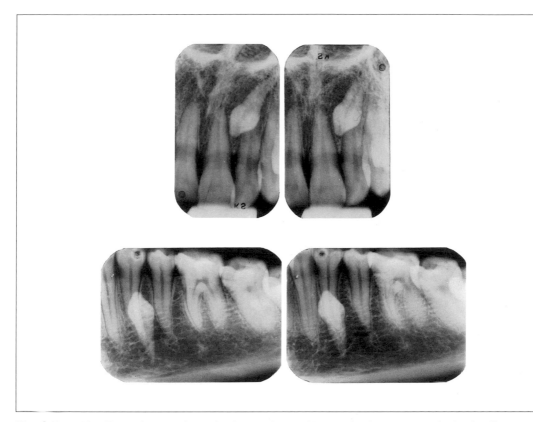

Figs. 2-6a and b   Two pairs or radiographs that can be used to exercise the stereoscopic viewing illustrated in Fig. 2-5.

These last two methods are mentioned only to give a complete picture of the various available techniques.

Image quality

The clarity of details is influenced by the quality of the image. The factors determining the quality of the image are contrast and the lack of definition (unsharpness).

The contrast concerns the differences in blackening which occur in the image. Simply stated, contrast is determined mainly by the radiation quality.

Unsharpness deals with the transition of the blackening of two adjacent areas. If the border of a structure is depicted, the image on the film should show an abrupt change in the blackening when the borderline of the object is passed. In practice, the image will show a gradual change in blackening spread out over a certain distance, this distance being the unsharpness in the image of this borderline.

The unsharpness is affected by three different factors: *(1)* movement during exposure of the x-ray source, the patient, or the film, resulting in *motion unsharpness; (2)* the size of the focal spot and the distances from the focal spot to the object and from

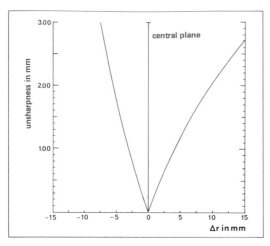

Fig. 2-7a   Increase of the unsharpness in the image of objects with increasing distance of the object from the central plane.

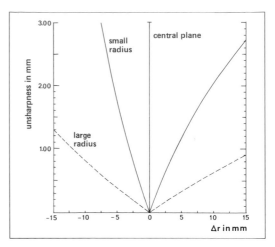

Fig. 2-7b   A smaller degree of unsharpness is produced when the distance of the central plane to the center of rotation is larger.

the object to the film, producing *geometric unsharpness; (3)* the diffusion of the projected image by the imaging medium, resulting in *recording unsharpness* (of special importance when intensifying screens are used).

In tomography and panoramic tomography, the latter of which is also called *rotational panoramic radiography,* only a layer that has a certain thickness (the *image layer)* within the patient is made visible. Objects outside this layer are made invisible on the film by producing motion unsharpness in the image of these objects. Fig. 2-7a shows how the unsharpness increases with the distance of the object from the plane, which is depicted without any motion unsharpness (this is the *central plane).* For a diagnosis that requires the visibility of small details (for instance, the shape of root canals) and therefore little unsharpness, only a rather thin layer is usable for the interpretation. If the diagnosis requires only the visibility of large struc-

tures (as for instance the presence of a tooth) a much thicker layer can be evaluated. The gradual increase of the unsharpness explains why it is impossible to give exact figures on the thickness of the layer that can be interpreted when the maximum acceptable unsharpness is not defined.

When the distance between the central plane and the rotation center (the radius) is small, then the unsharpness in the image will be large, and vice versa. This is graphically illustrated in Fig. 2-7b.

In most panoramic radiographic machines the distance from the rotation center to the central plane is small for the anterior area and large for the molar area (Fig. 2-8). As a result, the image layer is small for the anterior area and thicker for the lateral areas; this is illustrated in Fig. 2-8 by the shaded area. In machines like the Panorex, which use only two positions for the rotation center that are close to the molar area, this difference in imaging

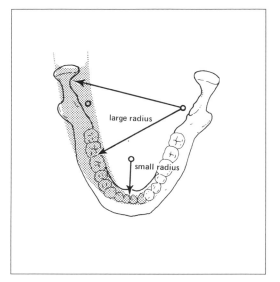

Fig. 2-8   The difference in thickness of the image layer for the different areas as a result of the different distances of the central plane from the center of rotation.

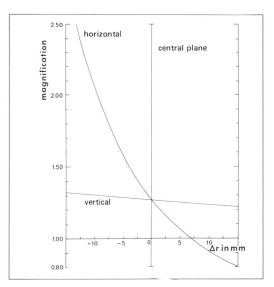

Fig. 2-9   The vertical and horizontal magnifications in the image are a function of the distance of the object from the central plane.

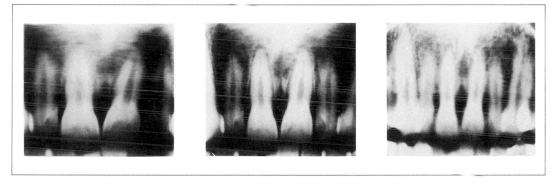

Fig. 2-10   Radiographs of the anterior area to show the effect on the image when different distances of the object from the central plane are used. The effects are caused by the difference in the unsharpness as well as the difference in the vertical and the horizontal magnifications (see Fig. 2-9). (A) the incisors 1 cm within the central plane; (B) the incisors at the central plane; (C) the incisors 1 cm outside the central plane.

quality between the different areas is less pronounced.

Another aspect of the image quality in panoramic radiography is the change in magnification of horizontal dimensions that occurs when an object is at a distance from the central plane. In the central plane the horizontal magnification is equal to the vertical magnification. Outside this plane there is only a negligible change in the vertical magnification; the horizontal magnification, however, increases rapidly toward the rotation center and decreases in the opposite direction (toward the film). This is quantitatively illustrated in Fig. 2-9. Figures 2-10a to c show the effect on a central incisor when the displacement is 1 cm. The size of an object may therefore be over- or underestimated when the object is not in the central plane.

The significance of different radiographic views for minor oral surgery in orthodontics

The aim of radiographic information is to detect deviations from normal anatomy for diagnostic purposes. The information specific for minor oral surgery can be classified as follows:
1. The presence or absence of normal and supernumerary teeth.
2. The presence or absence of a periodontal ligament and, if present, its width.
3. The mesiodistal angulation of a tooth.
4. The position of an impacted or supernumerary tooth relative to neighboring teeth.
5. The shape of the root and the crown of a tooth or a supernumerary tooth.

On the following pages, different radiographic views will be described and evaluated for their usefulness in studying the above-mentioned aspects.

In the descriptions no distinction will be made between a normal tooth and a supernumerary tooth; the term *tooth* will be used for both.

The following radiographic examinations will be evaluated:
1. Periapical examination
2. Occlusal examination
3. Lateral jaw examination
4. Panoramic tomographic examination
5. Panoramic radiographic examination using an intraoral x-ray tube
6. Lateral cephalometric examination
7. Posteroanterior cephalometric examination

Each type of examination is illustrated by radiographs to show the general appearance of the image and some examples to show their usefulness in diagnosing anomalies. Technical errors made in the production of the radiograph will not be discussed — a perfect technique is assumed.

The periapical examination (Figs. 2-11a to c)

For the periapical technique no-screen films are used. This results in images that show small details. Because of the size of the film used, the area shown covers only the teeth and closely surrounding tissues.

Presence or absence of a tooth

Because small details will be visible, this technique is very suitable for detecting unerupted teeth. It is, however, good to realize that other overlapping teeth can make the detection more difficult.

Presence / width of a periodontal ligament

Because small details will be visible, this technique is very suitable for evaluating the periodontal ligament.

Mesiodistal angulation of a tooth

The direction of the x-ray beam in this technique is often not parallel to the occlusal plane and at right angles to the dental arch. Thus, no accurate conclusions can be drawn as to the mesiodistal angulation of the tooth axis.

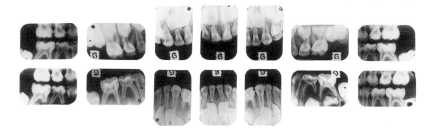

Fig. 2-11a A complete periapical examination of a patient with primary dentition.

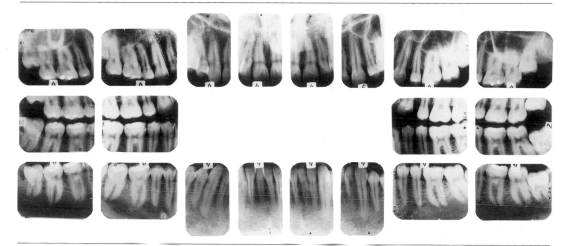

Fig. 2-11b A complete periapical examination of a patient with permanent dentition.

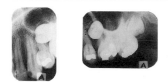

Fig. 2-11c A set of two films suitable for applying the AXIAL rule. Determine first the displacement of the x-ray tube and then find the position of the crown and the root of the impacted second premolar.

The only aspect that can be judged to any extent is a nonparallelism to adjacent teeth, provided there is no difference in the buccolingual angulation between these teeth. More reliable conclusions are possible when the right angle technique with an aiming device is used. A small film size (number 0 or 1) will be very useful to reduce the vertical angulation of the x-ray beam.

Position of an impacted tooth relative to neighboring teeth

When two views suitable for stereoscopic viewing are made, stereoscopic evaluation is possible. Two different views can be used for applying the AXIAL rule.

Tooth shape

Because small details will be visible, this technique is very suitable for evaluating the shape of a tooth.

The occlusal examination (Figs. 2-12a to d)

For this technique no-screen films are used. This results in images that show small details. In comparison with a periapical examination the vertical angulation of the x-ray beam is larger. Because of this increased angulation and the size of the film used, the images will show a larger section of the patient than in a periapical examination.

Presence or absence of a tooth

Because small details will be visible when an occlusal examination is made, this technique is very suitable for detecting unerupted teeth. It is good to realize, however, that other overlapping teeth can make the detection more difficult.

The larger area covered by the radiographs prevents the missing of impacted teeth at remote positions.

Presence / width of a periodontal ligament

Because small details will be visible, this technique is very suitable for evaluating the periodontal ligament.

Mesiodistal angulation of a tooth

Because the vertical angulation is intentionally large, this view is not suitable for evaluating the mesiodistal angulation of a tooth.

Position of an impacted tooth relative to neighboring teeth

When two views suitable for stereoscopic viewing are made, stereoscopic evaluation is possible. Two different views can be used for applying the AXIAL rule.

Occlusal views can be combined with a panoramic tomographic view to obtain information in two directions at right angles to each other, which facilitates the positioning of an unerupted tooth. For the anterior area this is possible by combining the occlusal view with either a lateral or a posteroanterior (P-A) cephalometric view.

Tooth shape

Because small details will be visible, this technique is very suitable for evaluating the shape of a tooth.

The lateral jaw examination (Figs. 2-13a to c)

For the lateral jaw technique, cassettes with screen-film combinations are generally used. This results in recording unsharpness, which will hamper the detection of small details. The ability to cover the lateral area of the maxilla and mandible on one film with the use of an extraorally positioned cassette is one of the advantages of this technique.

Presence or absence of a tooth

Because of the unsharpness, this technique is not suitable for detecting small de-

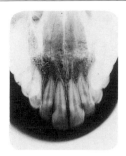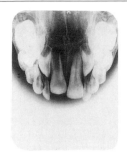

Fig. 2-12a   Two occlusal views of the maxillary anterior area of a patient, one with the permanent and one with the primary dentition.

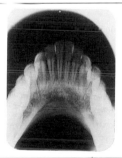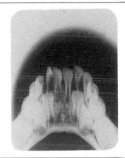

Fig. 2-12b   Two occlusal views of the maxillary lateral area of a patient, one with the permanent and one with the primary dentition.

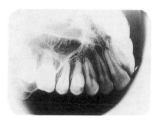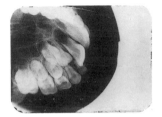

Fig. 2-12c   Two occlusal views of the mandibular anterior area of a patient, one with the permanent and one with the primary dentition. For the lateral area of the mandible, the lateral jaw examination is more appropriate.

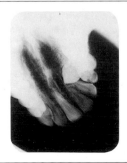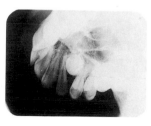

Fig. 2-12d   A set of two films suitable for applying the AXIAL rule. The displacement of the x-ray tube should be determined first.

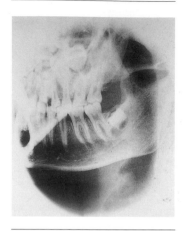 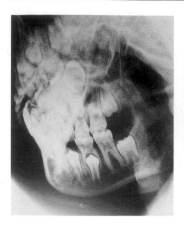 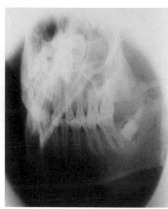

Fig. 2-13a   A lateral jaw examination of the mandible of a patient with a permanent dentition.

Figs. 2-13b and c   Two lateral jaw examinations depicting the lateral area of both the mandible and the maxilla. One image of a permanent and one of a primary dentition.

tails; however, teeth are generally large enough to be detected.

Presence / width of a periodontal ligament
Because of the unsharpness, periodontal ligaments, which are relatively narrow, may be difficult to find.

Mesiodistal angulation of a tooth
The direction of the x-ray beam is often not parallel to the occlusal plane and at right angles to the dental arch. Thus, no accurate conclusions can be drawn as to the mesiodistal angulation of the tooth axis.

The only aspect that can be judged to any extent is a nonparallelism with adjacent teeth, provided there is no difference in the buccolingual angulation between these teeth.

Position of an impacted tooth relative to neighboring teeth
In principle, two views can be used for a stereoscopic evaluation of the position of

impacted teeth. The freedom to change the angulation of the beam, however, is limited.

Tooth shape
Teeth are generally large enough for information to be collected concerning their shape.

The panoramic tomographic examination (Figs. 2-14a to c)

The panoramic tomographic examination will show only a predetermined curved layer of limited thickness that corresponds with the average shape of the dental arch. The unsharpness and the distortion in the image increase when the distance between the object and the central plane becomes larger.

Presence or absence of a tooth
Because of the image quality only objects close to the central plane can be visual-

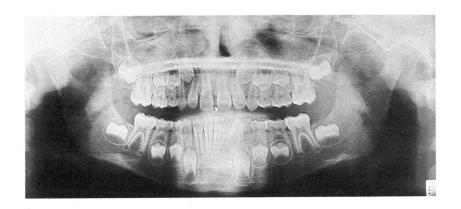

Fig. 2-14a Panoramic tomogram.

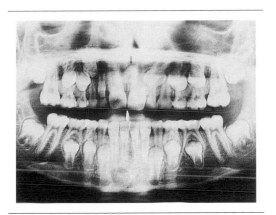

Fig. 2-14b Panoramic tomogram with an impacted tooth in the imaged plane *(arrow)*.

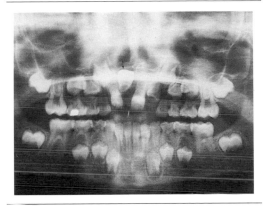

Fig. 2-14c Panoramic tomogram with an impacted tooth obscured because it is at a distance from the imaged plane *(arrow)*.

ized. Relatively large objects (complete teeth) can be recognized at a larger distance from the central plane.

Presence / width of a periodontal ligament

The periodontal ligament will only be visible when the tooth is close to the central plane. This is of special significance for the anterior area where the image layer is rather thin.

Mesiodistal angulation of a tooth

Because the direction of the beam makes only a small angle with the occlusal plane, the evaluation of the mesiodistal angulation of a tooth should be possible. The horizontal magnification increases rapidly and nonlinearly with a reduction of the distance of the object to the axis of rotation. As a result, the distance between teeth that are inclined with their apex lingually becomes larger toward the apex. When they are also inclined in a mesiodistal direction, curved roots are produced in the image. This effect is most pronounced in the anterior area. In the molar area the mesiodistal angulation can be estimated if the teeth are not extremely tilted in a buccolingual direction.

Position of an impacted tooth relative to neighboring teeth

Stereoscopic effects have been reported when two images of different layers are used, but this technique is not often practiced.

A panoramic tomographic view can be combined with an occlusal view to obtain information in two directions at right angles to each other, which allows the position of an unerupted tooth to be determined. For the anterior area, this is possible by combining a panoramic tomographic view with a lateral cephalometric view.

Tooth shape

Because of the unsharpness and the distortion as described for mesiodistal tooth angulation, this technique will give limited information.

The panoramic radiographic examination using an intraoral x-ray tube
(Figs. 2-15a to d)

There are two alternatives for this technique. In the first, the tube is positioned in the midline. Two exposures are required, one for the maxilla and one for the mandible. In the other technique, the tube is positioned between the occlusal surfaces of the molars on one side. The other side of the maxilla as well as the mandible are pro-

jected on one film. This technique requires two exposures, one for each side.

The midline technique produces images with large differences in the magnification for the different areas. Overlapping of teeth is unavoidable. These disadvantages are eliminated to a large extent in the lateral technique.

The area covered with both methods is much larger than with the intraoral technique. Exposures made on no-screen films will have approximately the same detail visibility as with the intraoral technique.

Presence or absence of a tooth

Because small details will be visible, this technique is very suitable for the detection of unerupted teeth. The large area covered is another advantage in this respect.

Presence / width of a periodontal ligament

Because small details will be visible, this technique is very suitable for evaluating the periodontal ligament.

Mesiodistal angulation of a tooth

Because of the short distance between the focal spot and the object, the projecting rays diverge greatly. This prohibits the evaluation of the mesiodistal angulation of a tooth.

Position of an impacted tooth relative to neighboring teeth

Stereoscopic images may be possible, but this has never been evaluated.

Tooth shape

Because small details will be visible, this technique is very suitable for evaluating the shape of a tooth.

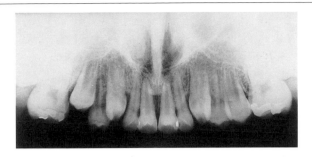

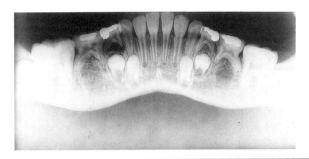

Fig. 2-15a   Image of the maxilla and one of the mandible obtained with the midline technique.

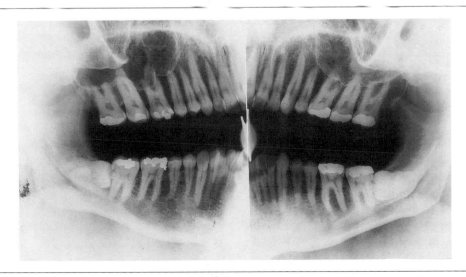

Fig. 2-15b   Two images obtained with the lateral technique, one of the right side and one of the left side of the patient.

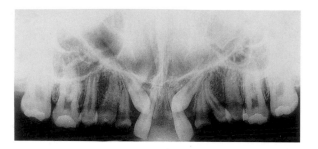

Fig. 2-15c   Patient with two impacted malpositioned maxillary canines. Image obtained using the midline technique.

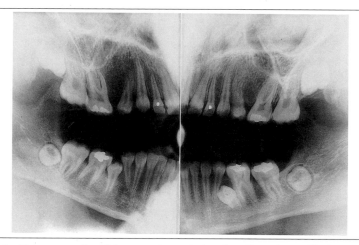

Fig. 2-15d   Patient with, among other things, an impacted malpositioned mandibular premolar. Image obtained using the lateral technique.

The lateral cephalometric examination (Figs. 2-16a and b)

In the lateral cephalometric examination, exposures are made on screen-film combinations. This reduces the detail visibility. Left and right sides of the dental arch are superimposed; this makes it difficult to separate the information from left and right.

Presence or absence of a tooth

Because of the overlapping of left and right, this technique can only be used to evaluate the anterior area.

Presence / width of a periodontal ligament

Because of the unsharpness, periodontal ligaments, which are relatively narrow, may be difficult to find.

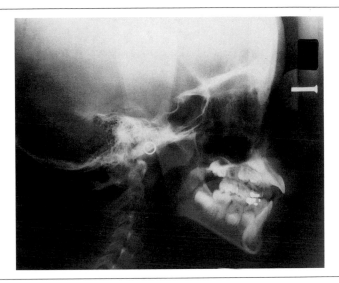

Fig. 2-16a   Lateral cephalometric view.

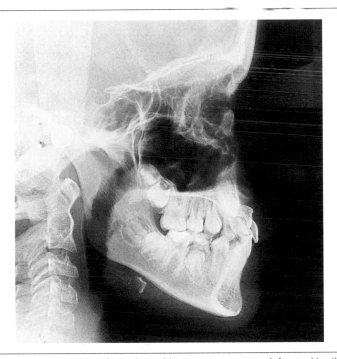

Fig. 2-16b   Lateral cephalometric view of a patient with a supernumerary deformed tooth in the anterior area.

Mesiodistal angulation of a tooth

Because of the direction of the projecting rays the evaluation of the angulation of teeth in the lateral area is possible if the overlap permits.

Position of an impacted tooth relative to neighboring teeth

Stereoscoping views are possible only when the strict rules for a cephalometric projection are ignored.

For the anterior area, the lateral cephalometric view can be combined with either an occlusal view, a panoramic tomographic view, or a posteroanterior cephalometric view to obtain information in two directions at right angles to each other.

Tooth shape

Because of the overlapping in the lateral area, only a tooth in the anterior area can be evaluated.

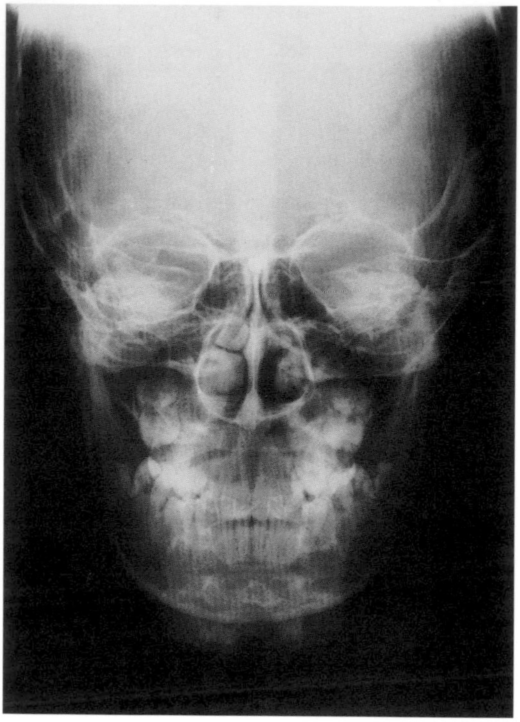

Fig. 2-17   Posteroanterior cephalometric view.

The posteroanterior cephalometric examination (Fig. 2-17)

Exposures made with the posteroanterior technique are made on screen-film combinations, reducing the detail visibility. The teeth in each lateral area of the dental arch are superimposed. This makes it difficult to collect information from the lateral areas.

The cervical vertebrae are projected over the anterior area, which hinders the interpretation of this area.

Presence or absence of a tooth

Overlapping structures render this technique unsuitable for detecting teeth.

Presence / width of a periodontal ligament

Again, the overlapping structures, as well as the use of intensifying screens, make this technique unsuitable in this situation.

Mesiodistal angulation of a tooth

Only the anterior area can be used to evaluate tooth angulations, because of the direction of the x-ray beam.

Position of an impacted tooth relative to neighboring teeth

Stereoscopic views are possible only when the strict rules for a cephalometric projection are ignored.

When the superimposition of the cervical vertebrae permits, it is possible to com-

Table 2-1   Suitability of seven radiographic evaluation types for use in various data

| Type of examination | Aspects of a tooth to be examined: | | | | |
	Presence	Periodontal ligament	Mesiodistal angulation	Position	Shape
Periapical	+	+	– (+)	+	+
Occlusal	+	+	–	ff + +	+
Lateral jaw	+ –	+ –	–	–	+ –
Panoramic tomography	+ –	–	+ –	f + –	+ –
Panoramic intraoral	+	+	–	–	+
Lateral cephalograph	– fr+	–	–	fff –	–
Posteroanterior cephalograph	– fr+	–	– fr+	f f –	–

+   = information can be obtained.
–   = information cannot be obtained.
+ – = information cannot always be obtained or only in specific areas.
fr+ = information can only be obtained for the anterior area.
+
|
+   = combination of the two techniques indicated with the + can give the information.
f
|
f   = combination of the two techniques indicated with the f can give the information for the anterior area.

bine the image of the anterior area of the dental arch in the P-A cephalometric view with either an occlusal view or a lateral cephalometric view in order to obtain information in two directions at right angles to each other.

Tooth shape
Because of the overlap in the lateral area, only a tooth in the anterior area can be evaluated.

Conclusions

Table 1 summarizes – the suitability of each technique in evaluating the different applications discussed.

Chapter 3

Congenital Absence of Permanent Teeth: Orthodontic Treatment Planning Considerations

Donald R. Joondeph

The congenital absence of permanent teeth introduces an imbalance in potential maxillary and mandibular arch length in the permanent dentition. Elimination of this arch length imbalance after complete eruption of the permanent dentition necessitates formulation of a comprehensive treatment plan that considers the possibility of orthodontic treatment, restorative treatment, or occasionally, a combination of the two. In most instances, an orthodontic approach would involve closure of the space created by the congenitally absent permanent tooth. A restorative approach would have as its objective the reestablishment of occlusal integrity by means of prosthetic replacement.

Congenitally absent maxillary lateral incisors

In situations where maxillary lateral incisors are congenitally absent, the choice between these two modes of treatment should not be made empirically. In most instances the presence or absence of major malocclusion symptoms serves as the primary criterion for either space opening or space closure. For a limited number of cases in which either treatment plan has the potential to provide an acceptable result, certain secondary criteria should determine the treatment approach.

Space closure

Lateral incisor spaces should be closed in cases with major malocclusion symptoms that require the extraction of permanent mandibular teeth. Mandibular extractions may be indicated to relieve either an anteroposterior arch length deficiency, to reduce a mandibular dentoalveolar protrusion, or to compensate for a Class II molar relationship. The choice of teeth for extraction should be determined by the location of the arch length deficiency, the amount of desired reduction in dental protrusion, and the anchorage requirements for molar relationship correction. Mandibular first or second premolar extractions are most commonly indicated. Less frequently, in order to compensate for intermaxillary tooth size imbalance or to avoid mandibular intercuspid width expansion, extraction of the mandibular incisor(s) is indicated.

Treatment planning for all cases in which

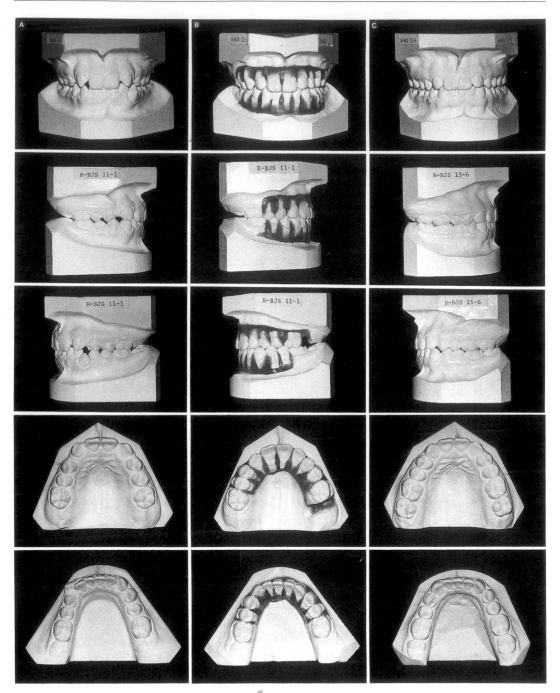

Fig. 3-1 *(A)* Initial study casts for patient aged 11 years, 1 month.
Fig. 3-1 *(B)* Diagnostic setup.
Fig. 3-1 *(C)* Final study casts for patient at age 15 years, 6 months.

maxillary lateral incisor space closure is being considered should include a trial diagnostic setup to determine the mandibular extraction combination that will provide the optimum functional and esthetic result. In addition, the trial setup will allow identification of tooth surfaces that require functional and esthetic reduction so that equilibration may be initiated prior to any necessary appliance placement.

Fig. 3-1 *(A)* shows a patient with congenitally absent maxillary lateral incisors and mandibular arch length deficiency, which requires extraction in the mandibular arch. The patient is an 11-year, 1-month-old girl with a mandibular anterior arch length deficiency and Class I molar relationship. A mandibular left lateral incisor extraction was indicated in order to relieve the mandibular arch length deficiency as well as to compensate for the interarch tooth size discrepancy. A favorable tooth size balance established by this combination of extraction and maxillary space closure is reflected in the pretreatment diagnostic setup (Fig. 3-1, *B*) and in the occlusal relationship following active therapy at 15½ years of age (Fig. 3-1, *C*).

Maxillary lateral incisor space closure is also indicated in certain instances not requiring mandibular tooth extraction. In cases with an end-to-end or Class II molar relationship it may be desirable to move the maxillary canines into the lateral incisor spaces and to establish or maintain the buccal disto-occlusion. Fig. 3-2, *A* illustrates the pretreatment casts of a 12-year, 9-month-old girl with congenitally absent maxillary lateral incisors, retained maxillary primary canines and right lateral incisor, and a Class II buccal occlusion. The absence of a mandibular arch length deficiency precluded mandibular tooth extrac-

tion, and the treatment of choice was to close maxillary lateral incisor spaces, treating to a Class II molar relationship. Fig. 3-2, *B* shows the final study casts, at 16 years, 4 months of age. This treatment plan is particularly expedient in postadolescent patients, in whom minimal mandibular growth potential limits the possibility of orthodontic correction of skeletal Class II relationships to either space closure or non-extraction tooth alignment in combination with orthognathic surgery.

Space opening

The absence of malocclusion symptoms requiring mandibular tooth extraction in combination with a Class I buccal occlusion generally favors treatment by orthodontic space opening and subsequent prosthetic lateral incisor replacement. Mandibular tooth extraction in these cases simply to compensate for closure of maxillary lateral incisor spaces may iatrogenically compromise facial esthetics and periodontal health or contribute to root resorption by the amount of tooth movement required to close residual spaces. Fig. 3-3 illustrates such a case. This patient had a Class I buccal occlusion, no mandibular arch length deficiency, and considerable excess space in the maxillary arch. Orthodontic treatment should be planned to maintain the buccal Class I relationship while retracting maxillary canines into a proper functional relationship. Maxillary lateral incisor spaces should be symmetrically created for future prosthetic replacement. These same criteria should be utilized to diagnose and plan the treatment of cases in the mixed dentition.

Fig. 3-4 illustrates a 9-year, 3-month-old

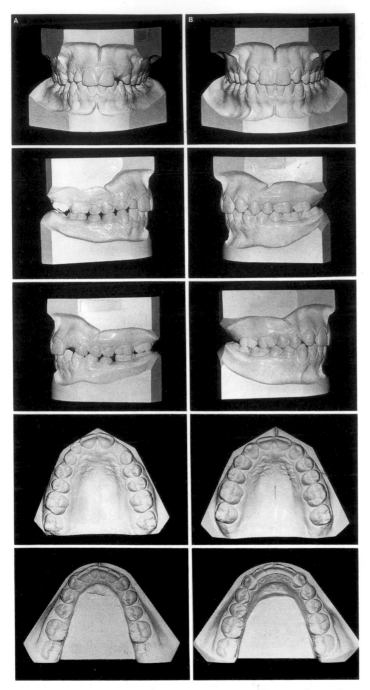

Fig. 3-2 *(A)*   Initial study casts for patient aged 12 years, 9 months.
Fig. 3-2 *(B)*   Final study casts for patient at age 16 years, 4 months.

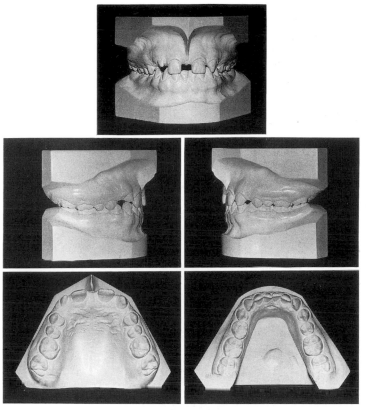

Fig. 3 3   Initial study casts for patient aged 13 years, 4 months.

girl who is congenitally absent both maxillary lateral incisors. She also has a Class I buccal occlusion with no maxillary and mandibular arch length deficiencies. A first phase of therapy is indicated at this time to close her maxillary midline diastema, allowing fabrication of an interim maxillary retainer, which will allow temporary prosthetic replacement of the missing lateral incisors. Maxillary primary canines should also be removed to encourage distal eruption of the permanent canines into a more ideal position. In planning either space closure or opening interceptively in the mixed dentition, it is advantageous to guide the permanent canines as close as possible to their final position to allow canine eminence development in that position and to improve treatment stability.

Secondary considerations in treatment planning

In cases where the major malocclusion symptoms do not definitively dictate either space opening or space closure, the clinician must rely on certain morphologic and functional criteria to determine the most favorable treatment approach.

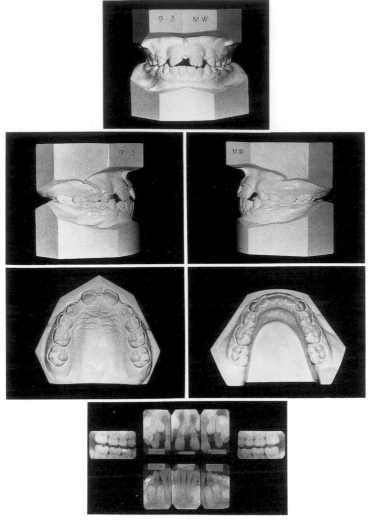

Fig. 3-4   Initial study casts and periapical radiographs for patient aged 9 years, 3 months.

Canine color

Substitution of canines for maxillary lateral incisors requires that canine color be compatible with the color of both adjacent and opposing teeth. Careful examination of color balance between canines and maxillary central incisors as well as canines and mandibular incisors may reveal a color incompatibility that would contraindicate lateral incisor space closure.

Additionally, when considering space closure one must account for the diminished translucency and darker canine color resulting from esthetic and functional recontouring of the canine incisal edge. If all other factors dictate lateral incisor space closure in spite of canine color incompatibility, incisal edge reduction should be minimized. Similarly, reduction of labial enamel may alter the color gradation of the canine as well as accentuate color differences between the canine and adjacent and opposing teeth. Canine — central incisor color differences may be more acceptable in males than in females and less apparent in individuals with darker complexions. Bonding and veneering techniques have added significantly to the clinician's ability to modify and harmonize these color differences.

Maxillary lip length

The esthetic impact of variations in tooth color and tooth shape is determined by the amount of tooth exposure during lip function. Thus, in patients with a relatively long upper lip, space closure may be acceptable in spite of major canine — central incisor color disparity. Conversely, in patients with a relatively short lip or with marked lip lifting during function, canine color incompatibility may contraindicate lateral incisor space closure.

Tooth size relationships

With closure of maxillary lateral incisor spaces, the most ideal esthetic balance will be achieved if canines are narrow mesiodistally relative to central incisors. However, if maxillary canines are relatively large, an acceptable esthetic result may be achieved through proximal canine reduction. Canines with convex surfaces and with thick proximal enamel lend themselves more readily to mesiodistal reduction than do canines with relatively flat con-

tours and thin proximal enamel. Caution should be exercised in reducing canine width mechanically because this may create difficulty in maintaining space closure in this area.

Perhaps more important than the esthetic aspects of tooth size relationships are the functional considerations. The replacement of lateral incisors with canines usually creates a maxillary anterior tooth size excess. The extent of this interarch imbalance can be detected through a modified Bolton's analysis. Possible methods of treatment compensation for this excess should be evaluated by means of a trial diagnostic set-up. Cases in the mixed dentition that require mandibular tooth extractions are more difficult to diagnose and treat because the lack of erupted permanent teeth makes it difficult to define the extent and location of the tooth size imbalance. It may be advisable in these instances to delay the extraction decision until sufficient eruption has occurred to allow a proper tooth size evaluation through a Bolton tooth size analysis and trial diagnostic set-up.

Canine position

The choice between lateral incisor space opening or space closure will also be influenced by the position the canines assume upon eruption. Instances in which canines erupt in close proximity to central incisors are best treated by space closure. The extensive distal bodily movement of such mesially positioned canines is not only mechanically difficult but is limited by the relative alveolar concavity between the canine and first premolar roots. This concavity is located in the area normally occupied by the canine root and accompanying canine eminence and may limit the achievement of ideal labial root prominence of the canine.

The clinician must weight these secondary criteria against one another and against the major malocclusion symptoms of arch length deficiency, dentoalveolar protrusion, facial esthetics, and molar relationship in order to arrive at the best possible treatment approach.

Occlusal function and equilibration with space closure

The substitution of canines for lateral incisors drastically modifies the functional occlusion. Because maxillary and mandibular canines do not occlude with each other, there is no potential for a "canine rise" occlusion during mandibular working excursions. The maxillary first premolars, mandibular lateral incisors, and maxillary and mandibular molars are most vulnerable to occlusal overloading under these circumstances. To preclude periodontal breakdown resulting from such overloading, proper occlusal equilibration is necessary. The objectives of occlusal equilibration should be:

1. To eliminate premature contact with the mandibular lateral incisors during working excursions by reduction of the maxillary canine incisal edge and lingual contour
2. To develop group function or modified group function in order to more evenly distribute the occlusal loads during lateral excursions, thus preventing first premolar overloading
3. To eliminate cross-tooth balancing interferences through equilibration of the lingual cusps of the maxillary first premolars; mesial rotation of maxillary first premolars for esthetic purposes will usually increase the potential for this type of interference
4. To eliminate cross-arch balancing interferences, particularly by equilibration of maxillary first and second molar lingual cusps

Occlusal equilibration is best handled in the following three stages:

1. Using the pretreatment diagnostic set-up as a guide, certain teeth may be reduced prior to appliance placement. Maxillary canines are best recontoured at this stage for establishment of proper tooth size relationship and centric occlusal contact with mandibular lateral incisors. Additionally, maxillary first premolar equilibration at this stage will allow the desired amount of mesial rotation for esthetic purposes without introducing cross-tooth interferences. Gross posterior interferences in centric occlusion may also be eliminated at this time.
2. Immediately following appliance removal, equilibration should be directed toward preliminary establishment of group function and elimination of major balancing interferences. Additional esthetic recontouring may be indicated at this stage.
3. After a period of retention and occlusal "settling," detailed functional equilibration should be accomplished.

By careful, sequential occlusal equilibration it is possible to establish an acceptable functional relationship even in the absence of normal canine position. Lateral incisor space opening with prosthetic replacement to achieve a canine-protected occlusion is seldom justifiable when most other treatment planning considerations indicate that space closure is preferable.

Summary

In cases of congenitally absent maxillary lateral incisors, the presence of major malocclusion symptoms usually dictates the choice between space opening for prosthetic lateral incisor replacement and space closure with canine substitution for the missing lateral incisor. In situations in which either treatment plan is feasible, the choice should be based on evaluation of certain secondary criteria, including acceptability of the resulting functional occlusion.

Congenitally absent second premolars

The congenital absence of maxillary second premolars also introduces an imbalance in potential maxillary and mandibular dental arch length in the permanent dentition. Elimination of this imbalance necessitates a comprehensive treatment plan that considers the possibility of orthodontic treatment, restorative treatment or, occasionally, a combination of the two. In most instances an orthodontic approach would involve closure of the second premolar spaces, whereas a restorative approach would have as its objective reestablishment of occlusal integrity by means of prosthetic replacement of the second premolars.

In selected cases, retention of primary second molars as substitutes for absent second premolars offers a third solution. This course of treatment is predicated on the presence of sound nonresorbing, non-ankylosed primary second molar roots and on the absence of a malocclusion for which active orthodontic correction is otherwise indicated. Under these circumstances, the attainment of satisfactory occlusal interdigitation may require proximal reduction of the retained primary molars in order to bring their mesiodistal dimension closer to that of a normal second premolar.

Orthodontic treatment of a patient with congenital absence of a second premolar and a completely erupted permanent dentition is dictated by the presence also of a malocclusion. Arch-length-deficiency malocclusions and Angle Class II malocclusions can be effectively treated by using the space created by loss or removal of the primary second molars for alignment of the remaining mandibular permanent teeth or for correction of molar disto-occlusion.

The most obvious advantage of orthodontic closure of such second premolar spaces over prosthetic replacement is the avoidance of abutment preparation of sound first molars and first premolars. A secondary advantage that may result from mesial movement of first and second permanent molars is creation of additional space for mandibular third molars, which otherwise may not be accommodated in the dental arch. On the other hand, closure of second premolar spaces and establishment of root parallelism between first molars and first premolars is a difficult and time-consuming manipulation if treatment is deferred until the permanent dentition completely erupts.

Loss of molar-premolar contact relationship and an increase in the curve of Spee

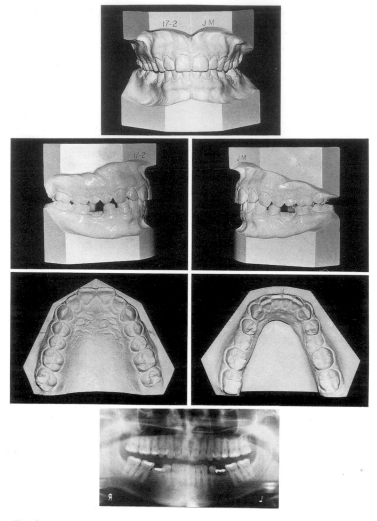

Fig. 3-5 Initial study casts and panoramic radiograph for patient aged 17 years, 2 months.

due to inability to maintain root parallelism are common postretention sequelae of this form of treatment. Fig. 3-5 illustrates a case in which a 17-year, 2-month-old boy has complete permanent tooth eruption and both mandibular second premolars are congenitally absent. A Class I buccal occlusion in combination with lack of maxillary and mandibular arch length deficien-cies preclude the ability to treat via orthodontic space closure. Resorbing primary second molar roots make further retention of these teeth unlikely. Additionally, both primary second molars are ankylosed, which has allowed tipping of the adjacent first molars and first premolars over the ankylosed primary molars.

Vertical eruption of the opposing maxillary premolar is in the initial stages, and treatment should be undertaken as soon as possible to avoid irreversible vertical alveolar development. The treatment plan of choice for this individual is removal of both primary second molars in combination with nonextraction tooth alignment and arch coordination in preparation for prosthetic replacement of the congenitally absent premolars.

The possibility exists that properly timed interceptive measures instituted before the permanent dentition erupts will preclude the need for prosthetic replacement, reduce or eliminate the necessity for extensive orthodontic appliance therapy and minimize the undesirable postretention sequelae previously discussed. Mathews[1] has suggested that distal eruption of developing first premolars may be encouraged by mechanical movement of the overlying primary first molar into the second premolar space. Two case reports support his contention that a satisfactory molar-premolar-canine axial relationship may be attained in this fashion. However, a course of orthodontic therapy with fixed appliances during the mixed dentition stage was used to achieve the desired result.

Case reports are presented here to suggest an alternative interceptive approach. In these instances, early extraction of primary second molars permitted sufficient autonomous adjustment of permanent first molars and erupting first premolars so that an acceptable occlusal relationship was achieved either without orthodontic appliance therapy or with a minimal period of treatment after eruption of the permanent dentition.

Case reports

Three cases involving the congenital absence of one or more mandibular second premolars are described. The treatment plan in each of these cases was based on the assumption that the patient would receive comprehensive orthodontic treatment after eruption of the permanent dentition. In each instance, however, the decision to forego full-appliance therapy was made by the patient. Partial appliances, which included cervical headgear, maxillary bite plate, or passive lingual arch, were used as indicated in the case reports.

Case 1 (Fig. 3-6)

This patient was a 9-year-old girl whose mandibular right second premolar was congenitally absent. Cephalometric and clinical evaluation revealed a Class I skeletal pattern, a Class II molar relationship on the right side due to premature loss of the primary second molar, and moderate mandibular arch length deficiency (Fig. 3-6, A). When the patient turned 9½ the maxillary and mandibular left primary second molars, the maxillary right and left first premolars, and the mandibular left second premolar were extracted. Appliance therapy with a maxillary cervical headgear and a maxillary bite plate was carried out for 4 months, after which the molars were in an over-corrected Class I relationship and the overbite was reduced. A maxillary retainer to maintain molar position was used until the patient reached the age of 11 years, 7 months. No mandibular appliances were used. Subsequent orthodontic records were taken at that time (Fig. 3-6, B) and at the age of 25 years, 7 months (Fig. 3-6, C).

Periapical radiographs of the patient are shown prior to primary molar extraction at age 9 years, 2 months (Fig. 3-6, D) and subsequent to autonomous space closure at age 27 years, 11 months (Fig. 3-6, E).

Fig. 3-6, F is a composite mandibular cephalometric tracing of the patient at 9 years (clear), 11 years, 7 months (solid), and at 25 years, 7 months (shaded). Note continued distal movement of the first premolar root after achievement of occlusal contact.

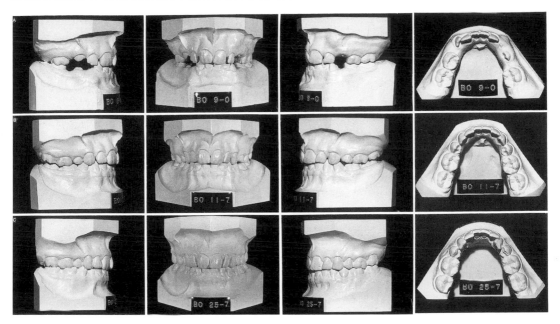

Fig. 3-6 *(A)* Initial study casts for patient aged 9 years.
Fig. 3-6 *(B)* Study casts at age 11 years, 7 months.
Fig. 3-6 *(C)* Study casts at age 25 years, 7 months.

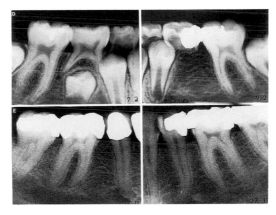

Fig. 3-6 *(D)* Periapical radiographs at age 9 years, 2 months.
Fig. 3-6 *(E)* Periapical radiographs at age 27 years, 11 months.

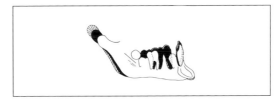

Fig. 3-6 *(F)* Mandibular cephalometric composite tracing.

Case 2 (Fig. 3-7)

The patient was an 8-year, 5-month-old girl whose mandibular right and left second premolars and maxillary right second premolar were congenitally absent. Cephalometric and clinical evaluation revealed a Class I skeletal and dental relationship with slight mandibular anterior arch length deficiency (Fig. 3-7, *A*).

All remaining primary teeth were extracted at this time with the exception of the maxillary left primary molars. Appliance therapy with a passive mandibular lingual arch and a maxillary bite plate was instituted 1 year later. The maxillary left primary first molar and first premolar were removed when the patient was 10 years, 5 months old, and appliances were discontinued 12 months later. Subsequent orthodontic study models were taken at the ages of 11 years, 7 months (Fig. 3-7, *B*), and 17 years, 7 months (Fig. 3-7, *C*).

Periapical radiographs of the patient are shown at 8 years, 2 months of age, prior to primary molar extraction (Fig. 3-7, *D*) and subsequent to autonomous space closure at age 17 years, 11 months (Fig. 3-7, *E*).

Fig. 3-7, *F* reveals a composite mandibular cephalometric tracing of the patient at age 8 years, 5 months *(clear)* and 17 years, 7 months *(solid)*.

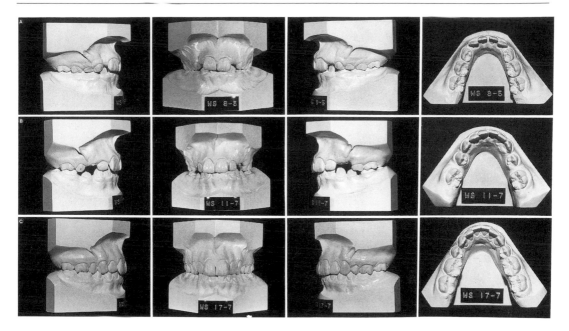

Fig. 3-7 *(A)*   Initial study casts for patient aged 8 years, 5 months.
Fig. 3-7 *(B)*   Study casts at age 11 years, 7 months.
Fig. 3-7 *(C)*   Study casts at age 17 years, 7 months.

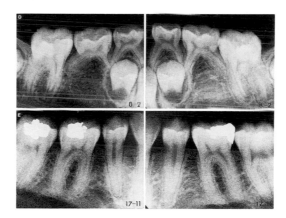

Fig. 3-7 *(D)*   Periapical radiographs at age 8 years, 2 months.
Fig. 3-7 *(E)*   Periapical radiographs at age 17 years, 11 months.

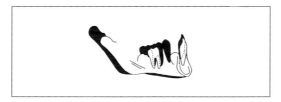

Fig. 3-7 *(F)*   Mandibular cephalometric composite tracing.

57

Case 3 (Fig. 3-8)

The patient was a 9-year, 9-month-old boy whose mandibular second premolars were congenitally absent. Cephalometric and clinical evaluation revealed a Class I skeletal pattern, a Class II molar relationship due to premature loss of primary second molars, and adequate mandibular dental arch length (Fig. 3-8, A).

Mandibular primary first and second molars were extracted when the patient was 10 years, 2 months of age. Appliance therapy consisting of a passive mandibular lingual arch and a maxillary bite plate with springs for correction of mesial molar tipping was instituted at 10 years, 3 months. Use of the lingual arch was discontinued at 12 years, 4 months, at which time the maxillary premolars were removed. The maxillary bite plate was continued as a retention appliance until the age of 13 years, 2 months. Orthodontic study models were taken at 12 years, 4 months (Fig. 3-8, B) and at 19 years, 11 months (Fig. 3-8, C).

Periapical radiographs of the patient are shown prior to primary molar extraction at 8 years, 5 months (Fig. 3-8, D), and subsequent to autonomous space closure at 17 years, 10 months (Fig. 3-8, E).

Fig. 3-8, F is a composite mandibular cephalometric tracing of the patient at 9 years, 9 months (clear), 12 years, 4 months (solid), and 19 years, 11 months (shaded). Note continued distal movement of first premolar root after achievement of occlusal contact.

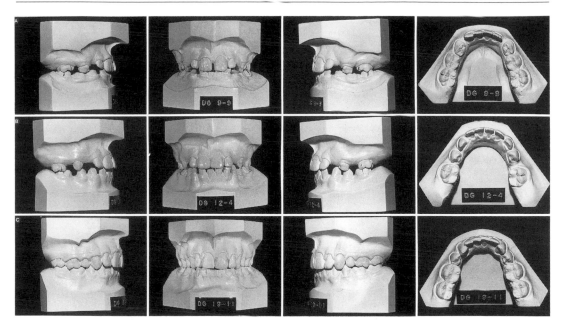

Fig. 3-8 *(A)*   Initial study casts for patient aged 9 years, 9 months.
Fig. 3-8 *(B)*   Study casts at age 12 years, 4 months.
Fig. 3-8 *(C)*   Study casts at age 19 years, 11 months.

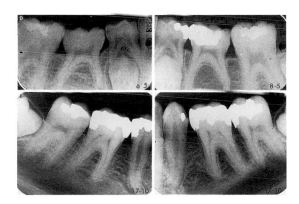

Fig. 3-8 *(D)*   Periapical radiographs at age 8 years, 5 months.
Fig. 3-8 *(E)*   Periapical radiographs at age 17 years, 10 months.

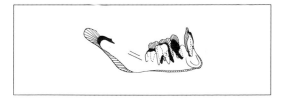

Fig. 3-8 *(F)*   Mandibular cephalometric composite tracing.

Discussion

The mechanistic orientation of orthodontic practitioners too frequently leads to the belief that tooth movements over long distances occur in a favorable fashion only if guided by active appliance therapy. Thus, the potential of autonomous tooth movement is often overlooked in planning treatment of malocclusions. The occasional correction of an arch length deficiency malocclusion solely by serial extraction and the frequent reduction of treatment complexities subsequent to serial extraction serve as testimony to the efficacy of noncontrolled tooth movement.

Extraction decisions in cases involving congenital absence of mandibular second premolars in the mixed dentition are based upon the same criteria applicable to cases involving a full complement of teeth. If a mandibular arch length deficiency exists or reduction of a dentofacial protrusion would require extraction of permanent teeth, early removal of primary second molars is indicated. Retention of primary second molars with eventual prosthetic replacement should be considered in cases with malocclusions not necessitating permanent tooth removal.

The timing of primary molar extraction and the pattern of tooth eruption play a major role in determining the potential development of a satisfactory occlusion autonomously. If maximum distal drift of first premolars is desirable in order to relieve mandibular incisor and canine crowding, primary second molars should be extracted at a time when the potential for distal drift is greatest, ie, while first premolars are still undergoing root development and active eruption, but prior to establishment of occlusion with their antagonists. The

exact time of primary second molar extraction within this developmental interval does not appear to be critical.

Satisfactory bodily drift was achieved with extraction times ranging from initial first premolar root development and minimal primary first molar root resorption (Figs. 3-7, *D* and 3-8, *D*) to two-thirds premolar root development and complete primary molar root resorption (Fig. 3-6, *E*). On the other hand, primary molar extraction must be deferred until one is certain that second premolars are, in fact, congenitally absent and not simply delayed in their calcification. Evaluation of first premolar root development and the degree of calcification of the remaining second premolars can be used as a guide in this respect. Riedel[2] believes that the earlier first and second primary molars are removed, the more satisfactory will be the resulting occlusion. He suggests primary molar extraction as soon as possible after permanent incisor eruption.

Acceptability of the autonomous space closure resulting from early primary second molar extraction is judged by the establishment of satisfactory contact relationship between first molar and premolar and the attainment of satisfactory axial root parallelism of teeth adjacent to the extraction site. Achievement of these objectives ensures that occlusal loads carried by the teeth are coincident with their long axes, that a proper marginal ridge relationship exists, and that there are no "triangular" interproximal spaces, which may be more susceptible to food impaction and future periodontal breakdown. Typically, in the first premolar serial extraction case, which does not undergo active appliance therapy, satisfactory root parallelism, and contact relationship are not autonomously

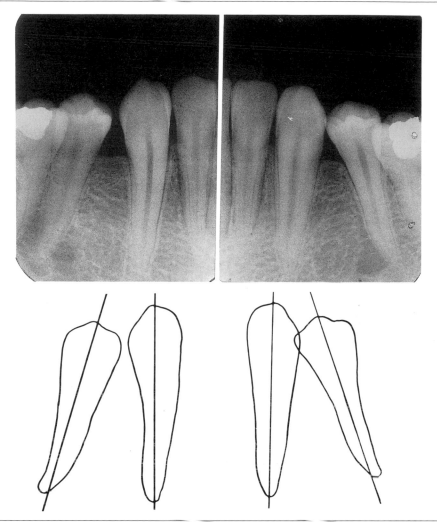

Fig. 3-9　Mandibular periapical radiographs and tracing of an untreated first premolar serial extraction.

achieved. In the mandibular arch, distal inclination of the canine and mesial inclination of the second premolar into the extraction site are the common result of this form of treatment (Fig. 3-9). Appliance therapy following first premolar serial extraction is generally directed at reducing this unfavorable axial and contact relationship in conjunction with leveling of the Curve of Spee.

Interestingly enough, in the cases presented in which second premolars were congenitally absent, root parallelism and contact relationship of first premolar and first molar were quite satisfactory following autonomous space closure of the second premolar area (Figs. 3-6, *E*, 3-7, *E*, 3-8, *E*, and 3-10). This relationship is due to bodily movement of the first molar and premolar

61

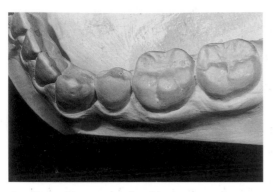

Fig. 3-10   Contact relationship between first premolar and first molar in the mandibular arch of an untreated patient in which second premolars were congenitally absent and space was allowed to draft autonomously.

into the second premolar space, as illustrated by mandibular serial cephalometric tracings superimposed on the mandibular synthesis and inferior alveolar nerve canals (Figs. 3-6, *F,* 3-7, *F,* and 3-8, *F*). The observed bodily migration is associated with limited lingual incisor movement and minimal increase in the Curve of Spee and incisor overbite. In the patient shown in Fig. 3-11, the Curve of Spee was actually reduced during autonomous space closure, and mandibular incisor inclination appears to have improved during this time.

Possible explanations for this space closure being achieved by bodily movement rather than by tipping include the capability for unrestricted molar and premolar root movement afforded by the absence of a second premolar bud and/or the provision of adequate space for distal migration of the first premolar during early stages of root development and eruption.

Summary

Orthodontic treatment in cases with congenitally absent second premolars and complete eruption of the permanent dentition is directed toward retention of the primary second molar, providing it is nonankylosed and nonresorbing and the concomitant tooth size discrepancy can be eliminated through interproximal tooth size reduction. Orthodontic space closure of the congenitally absent spaces should be considered in instances where extraction in the mandibular arch is indicated because of either a significant arch length deficiency, dentofacial protrusion, or Class II molar relationship. In situations where the patient presents with malocclusion symptoms that preclude space closure, the treatment should be directed toward orthodontic tooth alignment in preparation for prosthetic replacement of the congenitally absent teeth.

If cases with congenitally absent premolars are identified in the early stages, interceptive approaches may be instituted to avoid the extensive tooth movement required to close spaces once complete permanent tooth eruption has taken place. Early recognition and treatment plan formulation may allow interceptive extraction of primary molars. This early extraction procedure allows bodily space closure to occur autonomously and is associated with satisfactory root parallelism and contact relationship in the extraction site with minimal appliance therapy.

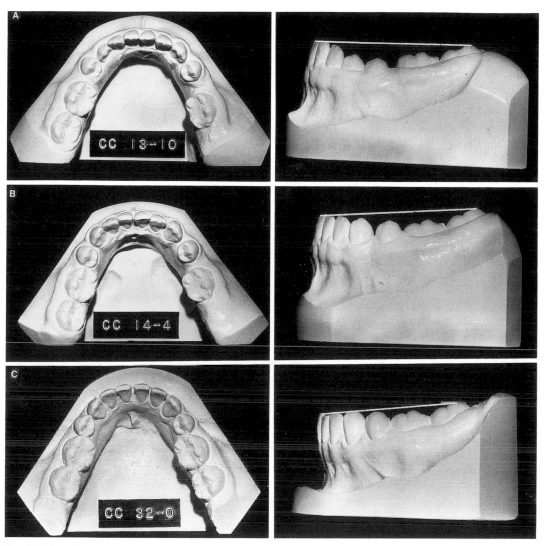

Fig. 3-11 *(A)* Study casts for patient aged 13 years, 10 months.
Fig. 3-11 *(B)* Study casts at age 14 years, 4 months.
Fig. 3-11 *(C)* Study casts at age 32 years.

References

1. *Mathews J:* Translation movement of first deciduous molars into second molar positions. *Am J
   Orthod* 1969; 55 : 276–285.
2. *Riedel R A:* Personal communication.

Chapter 4

Principles of Oral Surgery

Daniel M. Laskin

Although most discussions of the principles of surgery are generally concerned with factors that relate only to the operative procedure, such an approach neglects two very essential areas that can play an equally important role in determining surgical success or failure — adequate preoperative preparation of the patient and proper postoperative care. Therefore, while the greatest emphasis in this chapter will be placed on the intraoperative principles of oral surgery, these other factors will also be discussed in the light of how they can influence the operative results. This is essential because the most precisely executed operation can fail if a complicating medical condition has been overlooked or if the patient is either not given adequate postsurgical instructions or fails to heed them when they are provided.

Preoperative evaluation of the patient

One of the most frequently neglected aspects of surgical care is the preoperative evaluation of the patient. Proper attention to this matter can result in appropriate modifications in therapy, and this can avoid some of the more serious intraoperative and postoperative complications. There are three areas of major concern.

First, one needs to know about medical conditions that can complicate the surgical procedure. Impaired healing can occur in patients with anemia, certain vitamin deficiencies, diabetes, hypothyroidism, nephritis, and hepatitis; persistent bleeding can occur in patients with blood dyscrasias, hepatic disease, and vitamin C and K deficiencies; patients with diabetes, anemia, hepatic disease and hypoadrenalism are generally more susceptible to infections; and those with hepatic and renal disease may have inadequate detoxification or excretion of drugs.[1]

The second concern involves medical complications that can be caused by the surgical procedure. These include stress-related problems in diabetics or patients with heart disease or adrenal insufficiency; hemorrhage in patients with blood dyscrasias, and the consequences of bacteremia in patients with congenital or rheumatic heart disease.

Finally, there are concerns about patients taking systemic medications that can also complicate the surgical procedure.

For example, steroids can cause delayed healing and susceptibility to infection, and antihistamines and tranquilizing drugs can produce potentiation of analgesic drugs as well as sedation.

Both the history and the physical examination provide useful information about health status.[2] To obtain maximum information it is important to take a verbal history as well as to use a self-administered questionnaire.[3] When dealing with children, it may sometimes be necessary to question the parent as well as the patient, particularly regarding past history. When taking a history it is often helpful to begin with broad, leading questions and then focus on the specific areas of positive information that they elicit. Asking the following questions will be of value in bringing out a detailed history: *(1)* How is your general health? *(2)* Have you ever been or are you now under medical care and, if so, for what are you being treated? *(3)* Are you or have you been taking any medications? It is also important to obtain specific information about whether the patient has any congenital or organic heart disease, hypertension, diabetes, kidney or liver disease, as well as determine whether there is a history of rheumatic fever or a tendency to bleed excessively.

Although the limited physical examination performed by the dentist generally provides less information than the history, recording vital signs and examining exposed parts of the body can occasionally also provide information leading to the diagnosis of an unsuspected systemic disease.

When the presence of a systemic disorder is recognized, or the patient is taking medications that can lead to operative or postoperative complications, appropriate steps will need to be taken preoperatively to correct any deficiencies, alter the dosage of the systemic medications, modify the use or dosage of any drugs that will be employed in conjunction with the surgical procedure, and control the stress associated with fear and anxiety. Prophylactic antibiotics may also be necessary in certain patients to prevent bacteremia or infection[4] (Tables 1 and 2). It is frequently advisable to seek medical consultation when treating a medically compromised patient to ensure that all the necessary precautions are being taken.

The preoperative evaluation should not only include an appropriate history and physical examination but also a careful clinical and, often, a radiographic examination of the region of surgical interest. Failure to recognize the proximity of important anatomical structures, the presence of concomitant infection, or the association of other pathoses can only lead to perioperative and postoperative complications, most of which are otherwise avoidable. Proper radiographs need to be obtained when dental or osseous structures are involved. Generally, periapical views should be supplemented with panoramic radiographs and other views, depending on the particular problem, and these films should be carefully reviewed preoperatively.

Presurgical preparation of the patient

Because all operative procedures are physically and emotionally stressful, management of fear, anxiety, and pain is an important principle of surgical care. Such management should often begin with premedication on the night prior to the surgery so

Table 1 **Indications for prophylactic antibiotics**

Protection against bacteremia*	**Protection against infection +**
Rheumatic heart disease	Immunosuppression
Congenital heart disease	Severe debilitation
History of endocarditis	Postirradiation of jaws
Acquired valvular disease	Extensive trauma
Idiopathic hypertrophic subaortic stenosis	
Mitral valve prolapse with insufficiency	
Prosthetic heart valve	
Intravascular prosthesis, shunt	
Joint prosthesis ‡	

* Endocarditis prophylaxis is not indicated in patients with isolated secundum atrial septal defect, secundum atrial septal defect repaired without a patch 6 or more months earlier, patent ductus arteriosus ligated and divided 6 or more months earlier, or post — coronary artery bypass graft surgery.
+ No standard regimens exist. Antibiotics should be administered for at least 5 to 7 days.
‡ No standard regimen exists. Because opinions differ it is best to consult with the orthopedic surgeon prior to treating such patients.

Table 2 **Endocarditis prophylaxis for surgical patients***

Regimen	Patients	
Standard	Adults/Children over 27 kg	Children under 27 kg
Nonallergic to penicillin	2.0 g penicillin V orally 1 h before surgery and 1 g 6 h later; or 2 million units aqueous penicillin G intramuscularly 30–60 min before surgery and 1 million units 6 h late	Adult doses reduced by one half
Allergic to penicillin	1 g erythromycin orally 1 h before surgery and 500 mg 6 h later; or vancomycin 1.0 g intravenously slowly over 1 h, starting 1 h before surgery. No repeat dose needed	20 mg/kg erythromycin orally 1 h before surgery and 10 mg/kg 6 h later; or vancomycin 20 mg/kg given as in adults
Special+	Adults	Children
Nonallergic to penicillin	1.0 – 2.0 g ampicillin plus 1.5 mg/kg gentamicin intramuscularly or intravenously 30 min before surgery and 1.0 g penicillin V orally 6 h later	50 mg/kg ampicillin and 2.0 mg/kg gentamicin followed by 1.0 g penicillin V orally (500 mg for children under 27 kg) at same time intervals as for adults
Allergic to penicillin	1.0 g vancomycin intravenously given slowly over 1 h, starting 1 h before surgery; no repeat dose	20 mg/kg vancomycin as in adults

* Adapted from "A statement for health professionals by the Committee on Rheumatic Fever and Infective Endocarditis: Prevention and Treatment of Bacterial Endocarditis." *Circulation* 1984;70:1123A.

+ For patients at higher risk of infective endocarditis, such as those with prosthetic heart valves or with a previous history of endocarditis.

that the patient is able to sleep and therefore is better able to tolerate the stress of the operation. This is often particularly essential in the medically compromised patient, whose systemic condition can be severely aggravated by stress. Such patients should also be given morning appointments and should not be kept waiting, because anticipation of the procedure is often worse than the procedure itself.

Sedation during the operation is also an important aspect of stress management, as is adequate control of pain. Sedation also facilitates induction of anesthesia (local and general), produces amnesia, reduces oxygen requirements, and decreases the possibility of toxic reactions to local anesthetics. The choice of oral, rectal, parenteral, or inhalation sedation will depend on such factors as patient preference, age of the patient, degree of cooperation, duration of the procedure, and the medical status of the patient. These factors will also influence the choice of anesthetic agent. Although technically all of the surgical procedures related to orthodontics can be performed under local anesthesia, most patients are of an age that finds them highly uncooperative and difficult to sedate, and therefore the use of general anesthesia is often necessary.

The type of local anesthetic is generally determined by the medical status of the patient and the extent of the procedure. Because long-lasting anesthesia may be disconcerting to young patients, brief soft tissue procedures should be done with a short acting agent such as 2% procaine. On the other hand, longer procedures, with expectations of greater postoperative pain, should be done with longer-acting anesthetics such as lidocaine, mepivacaine, or bupivacaine.

Soft tissue procedures can usually be performed with an infiltration technique, which limits the area of anesthesia to the immediate surgical site. In young children, the less dense character of the bone also permits osseous surgery and exodontic procedures to be done with infiltration anesthesia. The disadvantage of the infiltration technique is that it may require multiple needle insertions. Although the pain can be eliminated by injecting into a previously anesthetized area, the idea of several injections may still be very frightening to the child. In such circumstances the use of a nerve block may be advisable. The discomfort of any anesthetic injection can be reduced by use of a topical anesthetic, sharp needles, distraction at the time of insertion, avoiding contact with the periosteum, injecting slowly, and avoiding the use of a cold solution.

The use of a vasoconstrictor in the local anesthetic solution prolongs its action and also provides hemostasis. Although the occasional episode of syncope seen in patients during injection of a local anesthetic has sometimes been blamed on the vasoconstrictor, most often it is related to fear and anxiety. However, the use of excessive concentrations of a vasoconstrictor can produce local tissue damage and postoperative pain in the injection site.[5] This can be avoided by limiting the concentration of epinephrine to 1:100,000 or 1:200,000, and using comparably low concentrations of levarterenol, levonordefrin, or phenylephrine.

The successful local anesthetic block depends on the use of an accurate technique, and attempts to flood the area with the anesthetic agent to compensate for a lack of such proficiency can only lead to undesirable complications. Generally, inability to consistently obtain anesthesia is due to use of a technique that is not based on stable, recognizable anatomic landmarks. Various reliable, anatomically based techniques have been described in the literature.[6] The same methods are used in adults and children; although the size of the structures is smaller in the child, the anatomic relationships are no different.

Failure to aspirate prior to injection of the local anesthetic can also be the reason for inadequate anesthesia in some cases. An intravascular injection not only dissipates the solution but also can result in toxic reactions to both the anesthetic and the vasoconstrictor. Proper aspiration, therefore, is an important principle to be observed in the use of local anesthetics.

The usefulness of prophylactic antibiotics prior to surgery to prevent postoperative infections in healthy patients has not been substantiated.[7,8] Their use preoperatively should therefore be limited mainly to patients with preexisting infection in the surgical site, immunosuppressed or debilitated patients, and those requiring specific protection against bacteremia[8,9] (Tables 1 and 2).

Steroids can be used prophylactically before surgery to limit postoperative edema in patients having extensive procedures.[10] Those steroids with the greatest glucocorticoid activity, such as dexamethasone, betamethasone, or methylprednisolone are the most potent antiinflammatory agents, and their use is therefore preferable to a full-spectrum corticosteroid such as hydrocortisone.

Asepsis

Because the mouth is a bacterially con-taminated cavity, there is sometimes a tendency to be unconcerned about sterility when performing surgery in the area. This is a serious mistake because not only can the surgical trauma reduce tissue resistance to infection from existing oral organisms, but also the tissues are normally susceptible to infection by organisms from other sources.[11] Therefore, every attempt must be made to operate in as aseptic a manner as possible. The perioral region should be cleansed with an iodophor compound or a hexachlorophene solution, and an antiseptic mouthrinse can also be used to reduce the oral flora and the potential for bacteremia.

All instruments must be carefully sterilized. Because protein and other polymolecular structures, particularly when dry, can serve as a protective covering for microorganisms and prevent penetration of sterilizing media,[12] instruments should be scrupulously cleaned of all blood, saliva, and necrotic material prior to sterilization. Although certain instruments that have small crevices, such as burs or bone files, need to be scrubbed by hand with a wire brush and a detergent, most instruments can be cleaned in an ultrasonic cleaning device.

Heat is the most effective method of sterilization. Heat may be transmitted through air (dry heat), water (boiling water or steam) or oil (hot oil). For those objects that may be damaged by heat, cold sterilization in a glutaraldehyde solution is very effective. It will kill bacteria, spores, and fungi, and even most viruses if given sufficient exposure.[13] When sterilized in glutaraldehyde, the instruments must be thoroughly rinsed in sterile water before use because the solution is toxic to living tissues.

Prior to surgery, the fingernails should be cleaned and the hands and arms scrubbed with a brush and soap or an idophor scrubbing solution for 3 to 5 minutes. The hands and arms should then be thoroughly rinsed, allowing the water to run from the fingertips toward the elbow. They are then dried with a sterile towel. Gloves should always be worn during surgery for protection of both the patient and the doctor.

Management of soft tissues

Anatomic considerations

Surgical danger areas

There are only a few major anatomic structures that one has to be concerned about when performing soft tissue surgery within the mouth: the large blood vessels in the palate, tongue, and the region of the mental foramen; the lingual and mental nerves; and the parotid and submandibular ducts.

Blood vessels. The oral tissues are highly vascular, with an excellent collateral circulation. Therefore, there is generally no need to worry about surgically interfering with blood supply and producing tissue necrosis when making intraoral incisions. The only concern is with excessive bleeding for inadvertently cutting a large artery or vein. Such vessels are found in the hard palate (anterior palatine artery), the tongue and floor of the mouth (lingual artery, ranine vein), and in the region of the mental foramen (mental artery). When possible, incisions should be planned to avoid cutting these vessels. Otherwise, they should be isolated and ligated before being cut. Cauterization is usually inadequate for controlling bleeding from these vessels, and its use increases the chance for secondary hemorrhage.

Sensory nerves. Although cutting minor sensory nerve branches during intraoral surgery causes no recognizable problem for the patient, injury to major sensory nerves results in a considerable area of paresthesia or anesthesia. This can occur during surgical procedures in the region of the mandibular canal (inferior alveolar nerve), the mental foramen (mental nerve), and in the floor of the mouth (lingual nerve). When it occurs in the former sites, the patient complains of numbness or altered sensation in half of the lower lip and chin; damage to the lingual nerve causes sensory changes on one side of the anterior two thirds of the tongue. Because of the frequent sensory stimulation of the lips and tongue, loss of sensitivity in these structures is extremely annoying to the patient. When work is being done near the mental or lingual nerve it should be isolated and retracted with an umbilical tape. Because traction alone can produce transient sensory deficit, the patient should always be warned about this as well as about the possibility of more permanent loss of sensation when surgery is contemplated in these regions. If the nerve is accidently cut, it can be repaired by microsurgery.

Salivary gland ducts. The location of the parotid and submandibular salivary gland ducts must be considered when the cheek or the floor of the mouth is being operated on. If cut, the duct can be anastomosed over a small polyethylene tube kept in place for 7 to 10 days.[14] A simpler procedure, however, is merely to leave the wound loosely sutured and allow the proximal end of the duct to create a new opening at that point. When incisions are made in the region of the parotid or submandibular ducts, even if they are not involved in the surgical procedure, care must be taken to avoid encompassing these structures with the sutures used to close the wound because this will cause obstruction of the gland.

Muscle pull on intraoral incisions

Generally, incisions should be made parallel to the direction of muscle pull. In the mouth this is only a consideration in the tongue and lips. In these structures, the incision should be made along the long axis, if possible. In the cheek, where one would think muscle pull should be an important factor, decussation of the buccinator fibers distributes tension relatively equally in all directions so that incisions can be made in any desired location.

In the lips, cosmetic considerations may sometimes make it necessary to violate the principle of parelleling incisions to the direction of muscle pull and vertical rather than horizontal incisions are used. If vertical incisions extend across the mucocutaneous junction, it is essential to suture skin to skin and mucous membrane to mucous membrane to produce an even lip line. A proper approximation is ensured by placing the first superficial suture precisely at the mucocutaneous junction.

Healing of oral soft tissues

One of the favorable factors with intraoral surgery besides the excellent resistance of the tissues to infection is the rate of wound repair. Studies have shown that the epithelial turnover in oral mucosa membranes is much quicker than in skin.[15] Clinically, this is reflected by a more rapid healing of surgical defects. This makes complete closure of oral wounds less important than for skin wounds.

Another problem occurring on the skin, but not with mucous membrane, is the formation of heavy scars or keloids. Intraoral wounds generally heal with minimal scarring. When scars do develop, they usually become quite pliable within a few months. From a cosmetic standpoint, the presence of scars within the oral cavity obviously is not a problem.

Although one might expect the presence of saliva to have an adverse effect on the healing of oral wounds, the reverse is actually true. The saliva not only has a cleansing action, but it also contains antibacterial substances that help prevent infection. Moreover, as demonstrated experimentally, moist wounds heal more rapidly than dry wounds.[16] The moist environment, however, does have an effect on treatment methods. Wounds produced by cauterization or electrocoagulation often have a tendency to become macerated. For this reason, excision of lesions with a scalpel or by electrosection is preferred.

The presence of saliva also influences the type of suture that should be used for final closure of intraoral wounds. Catgut sutures tend to become soft, and untie very readily. Nonresorbable monofilament sutures such as those made from nylon also untie easily. Silk sutures are able to hold a knot well and are well tolerated by the tissues. However, they do have a tendency to accumulate debris. They also absorb fluid and therefore have a wicking effect that can result in bacteria being carried into the tissues. Polyglycolic acid sutures are tolerated best by the oral tissues. Although they are a polyfilament suture similar to silk, experiments have shown that they have less tendency to transmit organisms into the tissues.[17] They tend to resorb slowly, however, and after a week can cause irritation and inflammation. They should therefore be removed in 5 to 7 days rather than be allowed to resorb.

Incisions and flap design

Because intraoral scars are not visible, the placement of incisions and flaps in this region is determined mainly by convenience, access, and avoidance of damage to major nerves and blood vessels. The surgical approach should be designed to provide maximum access with minimum trauma to the tissues. There are often several ways in which a surgical site can be approached, and the incision or flap design can be varied, provided that the basic principles are not violated.

Incisions can be made with either a scalpel or an electrosurgical knife. Electrosurgery works on the principle of heating the tissue sufficiently to boil the intracellular water and vaporize the tissue.[18] It has been shown that after 4 days wounds made with a scalpel are stronger and heal much faster because electrosurgery produces more necrosis and inflammation.[19] The advantage of using electrosurgery lies mainly in its ability to produce a relatively bloodless operative field. It is also useful in removing tissue, such as for exposure of a tooth or elimination of an operculum.

Because a flap is an area of tissue separated from its blood supply on at least two sides, the major principles of proper design involve maintenance of as adequate a remaining blood supply as possible (Fig. 4-1). This means that incisions should not transect major vessels but should be placed parallel to them; that the base of the flap should be as wide or wider than the apex; that the flap should not have sharp angles; and that the number of side inci-

Principles of Intraoral Flap Design
● Plan incisions to avoid cutting major nerves, blood vessels, and salivary gland ducts.
● Make flap large enough to provide adequate access.
● Make the base of the flap as wide or wider than the apex.
● Place all incisions so that they will be supported by untraumatized bone.
● Limit the number of vertical releasing incisions.
● Place vertical incisions between the teeth to avoid creating an uneven gingival margin.
● Avoid sharp angles on the flap.

Fig. 4-1

sions should be kept to a minimum. The most ideal flap is one developed from a single straight incision (envelope flap) because it separates the tissue from its blood supply only at its base and one edge. If access is still not adequate, the incision can either be extended or a side releasing incision can be made. A second side incision can also be made, when necessary, but it is generally inappropriate to start with a "trap door" flap because such a flap obtains its blood supply from only one edge and therefore is less likely to heal without complications.

Incisions for flaps should be placed far enough from the surgical site to ensure that the wound margins are located over sound bone. This prevents collapse of the flap and dehiscence of the wound when there is a bony defect and provides an improved base for development of the secondary blood supply to the tissues. If possible, incisions should not be made through an area of thinned mucosa, such as over a bony prominence or a root eminence, because such tissue already has a reduced blood supply. When a flap is to be made around the teeth, the incision should be made in the gingival crevice and the integrity of the interdental papillae should be maintained. When a releasing incision is made in the interdental region, however, the entire papilla should be included because an irregular gingival margin may occur if the flap does not heal at its original level. For the same esthetic reason, when a single-side releasing incision in the anterior part of the mouth is used, it should be made at the posterior end of the primary incision, when possible, even though this may violate the principle of reflecting a flap away from the operator to provide better access and visibility.

When a flap includes the mucosa and the periosteum, the incisions should be made through both layers directly down to bone. The flap should then be carefully elevated in one piece without damaging the periosteum, and gently retracted. The assistant must be cautious not to catch the flap constantly in the suction tip because this can traumatize the tissues and further impair the vascularity. When the surgery is completed, the flap should be returned to its original position, and the wound margins should be approximated with fine interrupted silk or polyglycolic acid sutures placed with a small curved cutting needle. Suturing holds the tissues against the bone, stops the accumulation of food and bacteria under the flap, and prevents postoperative hemorrhage.

The corners of the flap are generally sutured first, then the side incisions, and finally the main incision. With an envelope flap, the initial suture is placed in the center of the incision and then each half is sequentially divided with sutures until adequate approximation of the edges is obtained. The sutures should not be tied too tightly because this will cause tissue necrosis, and the knots should be placed away from the incision to prevent excessive irritation to the wound. Prior to closure of any incision, adequate hemostasis must be obtained to avoid hemorrhage and hematoma formation under the flap, and following wound closure any blood accumulated under the flap should be expressed. Mucosal sutures can usually be removed in 3 to 5 days. When being removed sutures should be cut at the level of the mucosa to avoid carrying contaminated material into the tissues.

Management of hard tissues

Tooth extraction

The first principle in the extraction of teeth involves adequate reflection of the gingiva from around the neck of the tooth so that it will not be traumatized during the surgical procedure. The second principle involves selection of the proper extraction forceps. Although there are many types available, the ideal forceps is one designed to provide a firm grasp on the tooth while at the same time permitting the beaks to be placed as far down on the root as possible. Generally, this can be achieved best with a slightly narrow-beaked instrument. An ideal forceps also has the beaks in a straight line with the handle; this permits the most efficient application and direction of forces. However, such a design does not permit the forceps to be used in the posterior part of the mouth; for this purpose, curves have to be introduced into the design. Still, the smaller the amount of curvature introduced, the closer the design approaches the ideal.

When a forceps is applied to a tooth the beaks should not only be placed as far apically as possible but also during the extraction they must be kept parallel to the long axis of the tooth. This directs the forces properly and reduces the chance of fracturing the root(s). During the extraction, forces should be applied judiciously, gradually expanding the socket toward the thinnest bony wall, and with as much rotational movement as possible to avoid fracturing the outer cortical plate. If the tooth is difficult to remove with a reasonable amount of force, expansion of the socket with an elevator or small chisel, reflection of a flap and removal of buccal or labial bone, or sectioning of the tooth if it is multirooted are all means of facilitating removal.

Elevators can also be used to remove teeth or roots. They are used in two ways: as a lever or a wedge.[20] In loosening or removing teeth or whole roots, the principle of the lever is generally applied, with the buccal cortical plate serving as the fulcrum. Root tips are removed by applying the wedge principle — two objects cannot occupy the same space at the same time. This procedure works best when the instrument is smaller than the root tip to be removed. Otherwise, attempting to force a large elevator into a small space may inadvertently displace the root into adjacent anatomic regions such as the mandibular canal, the maxillary sinus, or the sublingual or submandibular spaces. If a root cannot be dislodged from the socket easily, an open-view procedure, rather than more force, should be used.

Although elevators are extremely useful instruments, better control of forces and more subtle directional changes can be achieved by using a forceps. There is also less likelihood of traumatizing the adjacent gingiva and alveolar bone. The first rule regarding the use of elevators is therefore "Use a forceps first, if at all possible."

Removal of bone

Bone can be removed with rongeurs, chisels, or burs. The type of instrument is not as important as the fact that it must be sharp and that the bone is removed as atraumatically as possible. Rongeurs can be used to remove cancellous bone or small cortical prominences or exostoses. However, removal of dense cortical bone generally requires the use of burs or chisels. When a chisel is used to expose a tooth or root it is more efficient and less traumatic to remove the section of bone in one piece than to shave it away gradually. However, when shaving of the bone is desirable, the chisel should be used with the bevel against the bone rather than in the usual manner, which causes the edge to penetrate deeply rather than shave the surface.

Burs in a high-speed handpiece are a very efficient and accurate way to remove bone. A round bur is preferable to a fissure bur because it is easier to control and does not clog as readily. Whenever a bur is used, a coolant spray should be applied to the bone to prevent overheating. It has been shown that a temperature of 47 °C maintained for 1 minute is sufficient to produce bone necrosis.[21]

Debridement

Once the hard tissue surgery is completed, it is essential to properly cleanse the wound. The area should be thoroughly irrigated with a sterile saline solution, aspirated, and carefully examined for loose fragments of bone, tooth, or foreign material, which should be removed. Sharp bony edges should be excised with a rongeur and smoothed with a file or bur. When a rongeur is used, it should be applied with a cutting and not a twisting action to avoid fracturing the bone. After a final irrigation of the wound, the incision can be sutured.

Hemostasis

Proper hemostasis is another important principle of surgery. It begins preoperatively with the medical history and physical examination in an attempt to recognize any bleeding tendencies. If a problem is suspected, the patient should be subjected to the proper screening tests, including prothrombin time, partial thromboplastin time, bleeding time, a platelet count, and fibrinogen concentration.[22] In a patient with a bleeding problem, cooperation with a hematologist is necessary in planning any surgical procedure.

Intraoperatively, bleeding can be minimized by infiltrating the surgical site with a local anesthetic agent containing a vasoconstrictor before starting the procedure. The concentration of epinephrine in the solution should be no greater than 1:100,000 because higher concentrations can cause severe ischemia and possible tissue necrosis. Aspiration should be done prior to injection to avoid placing the solution intravascularly.

After the surgical procedure has been completed, bleeding should be controlled in both the bone and soft tissues. Gingival or mucosal bleeding is easily controlled by the use of sutures. Bleeding from vessels in muscle should be stopped with electrocoagulation or by clamping and tying them.

Suturing the mucoperiosteal flap over an area of osseous bleeding will usually only mask the problem and continued oozing under the flap will produce excessive swelling and hematoma formation. Bleeding from the bone should therefore be controlled directly by compressing the bone over the bleeding vessel, electrocoagulation, or by applying a small amount of sterile bone wax. Hemorrhage from an extraction socket can usually be stopped by suturing the overlying gingiva; the walls of the socket enable sufficient pressure to develop to tamponade the bleeding. When the gingival margins cannot be approximated, it may be necessary to place a resorbable packing in the socket, such as gelatin sponge or oxidized cellulose.

Postoperative care

The prevention of postoperative complications begins with proper preoperative evaluation of the patient and careful attention to surgical technique. However, inadequate postoperative care can often reverse what has been accomplished pre- and postoperatively and lead to an unsuccessful result. It is therefore essential not only to provide patients with proper postoperative instructions but also to emphasize the role they must play in precisely carrying out these instructions. With young patients it is particularly important to elicit the cooperation of the parents. Postoperative instructions should deal with pain, swelling, diet, and oral hygiene (Fig. 4-2).

Control of pain

Pain is probably the postoperative problem most feared by patients. Although a certain amount of postoperative pain is normal, it

Principles of Postoperative Care

- Adequately control pain by proper use of analgesics.
- Control swelling by use of pressure dressings, cryotherapy, and steriods, when appropriate. Use heat to eliminate any swelling that occurs.
- Maintain adequate fluid and dietary intake.
- Initiate proper oral hygiene and wound care.
- Prescribe prophylactic antibiotics when indicated (see Table 1).
- Provide verbal and written instructions regarding patient's role and responsibility in postoperative care.

Fig. 4-2

can be adequately controlled by the proper use of analgesics. There are three basic rules in the use of such drugs.[20] First, the drug should be administered before the pain begins and continued for a sufficient time to circumvent the painful period. Second, it is much more effective to control pain by using small doses of the drug at frequent intervals rather than large doses infrequently. Finally, because the amount of pain will vary with the surgical procedure, an analgesic sufficiently potent to control the expected pain should be prescribed. The instructions to the patient should state specifically when to take the drug, how much, and for how long.

Control of swelling

Swelling is not only disfiguring but also the tissue distention can stimulate pain receptors and increase the patient's discomfort. Swelling can be due to both a posttraumatic inflammatory response and to postsurgical bleeding. By paying close attention to intraoperative hemostasis the latter can usually be avoided.

Postoperative edema can be controlled in three ways: pressure dressings, use of cryotherapy, and pharmacologically. The simplest pressure dressing is a gauze pack placed over the intraoral surgical site and held firmly by attempting to occlude the teeth. Such pressure dressings are generally used for about 30 minutes to stop bleeding, but can be used for several hours to diminish swelling, when indicated. Extraoral pressure bandages can also be used to control postoperative swelling; they are usually left in place for 48 hours.

Ice packs are also helpful in controlling swelling. Their refrigerant action diminishes pain as well. They should be applied to the surgical site intermittently, 30 minutes on and 30 minutes off, because continuous application leads to the reverse hemodynamic effect and increases rather than decreases circulation. Intraorally, crushed ice can be used to keep the area cold. Cryotherapy should be used for only 24 to 48 hours, after which intermittent application of moist, hot packs should be applied to help increase circulation and eliminate whatever swelling has occurred. The use of steroids is the most effective way to control postoperative swelling.[23] Both oral and intramuscular administration have been recommended.[10, 24] Usually the drug is given either the night before and the day of surgery, or only the day of surgery. Such short-term use has no effect on wound healing, body defenses against infection, or adrenal function.[25]

Proper diet

The pain or discomfort accompanying chewing and swallowing following oral surgery makes normal dietary intake very difficult. Children, in particular, can become dehydrated very readily and healing can be impaired. It is important, therefore, that adequate attention be given to maintaining proper nutrition and fluid balance. Specific instructions should be given regarding the type and consistency of diet to be eaten. Soft, bland, nonchewy foods are tolerated best, and frequent small feedings are better than attempting to maintain a schedule of three meals daily. Immediately after surgery a clear liquid diet may be preferable for a few days.

Oral hygiene

Maintaining cleanliness of the wound is another important consideration in promoting conditions for proper healing. Starting 8 to 12 hours after surgery the mouth should be rinsed at least four times daily, particularly after eating, with a solution containing a half teaspoon of salt in a glass of warm water. Most proprietary mouth washes contain alcohol or other substances that can be irritating to the surgical site.[26] If hydrogen peroxide is to be used, it should be diluted to half strength with water.[27] In addition to rinsing, patients should be instructed, when possible, to brush their teeth as usual. The lips can be kept from drying by applying mineral oil, glycerine or petroleum jelly.

Summary

There are many ways in which the various oral surgery procedures can be performed and each has its advocates. What ultimately determines which procedure is best, or if several are equally as good, is their conformity to the basic surgical principles. This chapter has attempted to delineate these principles. It must be remembered that the preoperative evaluation and preparation of the patient, and the initiation of proper postoperative care are equally as important as the careful execution of the surgical procedure. Violation of the basic principles in any of these areas invites unnecessary problems and complications — adherence to them does not guarantee success, because there may be other unknown variables, but it certainly improves the chances significantly. Understanding the basic principles of surgery also helps in explaining failures when they occur. In this way, mistakes are not repeated and future care of patients is improved.

References

1. Lynch M A, Brightman V J, Greenberg M S. Burket's Oral Medicine. Philadelphia: J. B. Lippincott Co; 1984.
2. Trieger N, Goldblatt L. The art of history taking. J Oral Surg 1978; 36:118.
3. Scully C, Doyle D. Reliability of a self-administered questionnaire for screening medical problems in dentistry. Community Dent Oral Epidemiol 1983; 11:105.
4. Sonis S T, Fazio R C, Fang L. Principles and Practice of Oral Medicine. Philadelphia: W. B. Saunders Co; 1984.
5. Laskin D M. Diagnosis and treatment of complications associated with local anesthesia. Int Dent J 1984; 34:232.
6. Malamed S F. Handbook of Local Anesthesia. St. Louis: C.V. Mosby Co; 1980.
7. Paterson J A, Cardo A, Strategos G T. An examination of antibiotic prophylaxis in oral and maxillofacial surgery. J Oral Surg 1970; 28:753.
8. Zallen R D, Black S L. Antibiotic therapy in oral and maxillofacial surgery. J Oral Surg 1976; 38:349.
9. Little J W. The need for antibiotic coverage for dental treatment of patients with joint replacements. Oral Surg Oral Med Oral Pathol 1983; 55:20.

10. *Hooley J R, Hohl T H.* Use of steroids in the prevention of some complications after traumatic oral surgery. *J Oral Surg* 1974; 32:864.

11. *Krizek T J, Robson M C.* Evolution of quantitative bacteriology in wound management. *Am J Surg* 1975; 130:579.

12. *Lawrence C A, Block S S. Disinfection, Sterilization and Preservation.* Philadelphia: Lea and Febiger; 1968.

13. *Stonehill A A, Krop S, Borick P M.* Buffered glutaraldehyde – a new chemical sterilizing solution. *Am J Hosp Pharm* 1963; 20:458.

14. *Rankow R M, Polayes I M. Diseases of the Salivary Glands.* Philadelphia: W B Saunders Co; 1976.

15. *Cutright D E, Bauer H.* Cell renewal in the oral mucosa and skin of the rat. *Oral Surg Oral Med Oral Pathol* 1967; 23:249.

16. *Winter G D.* Movement of epidermal cells over the wound surface. In: Montagna W, Bellingham E (eds): *Advances in Biology of Skin.* New York: McMillan; 1964; 5:113–127.

17. *Lilly G E, Osbon D B, Hutchinson R A, Heflich R H.* Clinical and bacteriologic aspects of polyglycolic acid sutures. *J Oral Surg* 1973; 31:103.

18. *Glover J L.* The bovie: a new look at an enduring technology. *Am Coll Surg Bull* 1986; 71:4.

19. *Tipton W W, Garrick J G, Riggins R S.* Healing of electrosurgical and scalpel wounds in rabbits. *J Bone Joint Surg* 1975; 57-A:377.

20. *Laskin D M. Oral and Maxillofacial Surgery.* St. Louis: C.V. Mosby Co, 1985; 2: chap 1.

21. *Erickson R A, Albrektsson T.* Temperature threshold levels for heat-induced bone tissue injury. *J Prosthet Dent* 1983; 50:101.

22. *Zallen R D. Oral and Maxillofacial Surgery.* St. Louis: C.V. Mosby Co, 1980; 1: chap 14.

23. *Schaberg S J, Stutler C B, Edwards S M.* Effect of methylprednisolone on swelling after orthognathic surgery. *J Oral Maxillofac Surg* 1984; 42:356.

24. *Huffman G G.* Use of methylprednisolone sodium succinate to reduce post-operative edema after removal of impacted third molars. *J Oral Surg* 1977; 35:198.

25. *Hooley J R, Bradley P B, Haines M.* Plasma cortosal levels following short-term betamethasone therapy for oral surgical procedures. *Trans Int Conf Oral Surg* 1973; 4:188.

26. *Bassett C, Kallenberger A.* Influence of chlorhexidine rinsing on the healing of oral mucosa and osseous lesions. A histomorphometric study in experimental animals. *J Clin Periodontol* 1980; 7:443.

27. *Martin J H, Bishop J G, Guentherman R H, Dorfman H L:* Cellular response of gingiva to prolonged application of dilute hydrogen peroxide. *J Periodontol* 1968; 39:208.

Chapter 5

Anatomy and Morphology of the Periodontium

Robert L. Vanarsdall

Introduction

No attempt will be made to provide an in-depth description of the normal features of the different tissues of the periodontium. However, certain periodontal morphologic relationships must be understood before minor periodontal surgery procedures for orthodontic patients can be performed. This chapter will provide a very selective and brief review. Performing predictable, effective, minor gingival procedures requires an understanding of anatomic variations of child and adult patients that are not usually delineated in periodontal texts. Recognition of these morphologic relationships will point to solutions to gingival hyperplasia, mucogingival problems, certain types of decalcification, increased stability, and esthetic improvement for orthodontic patients during and after orthodontic treatment.

Gingival landmarks

The oral mucous membrane that covers the alveolar process and the cervical portion of the teeth is called the *gingiva*. The tissue has classically been labeled the *free* and the *attached* gingiva. Normal adult gingival margin is found on the enamel approximately 3 to 5 mm coronal to the cementoenamel junction (CEJ) (Fig. 5-1). The base of the sulcus is the coronal portion of the junctional epithelium, which attaches the gingival connective tissue to the enamel from the cementoenamel junction. This attachment in the adult is usually 2 to 3 mm, and the high cellular turnover rate allows it to replace itself every 6 to 7 days.[1] During tooth eruption, the reduced enamel epithelium is gradually transformed into junctional epithelium (Fig. 5-2).

The attached gingiva (keratinized) extends from the bottom of the gingival sulcus to the mucogingival junction or zone (Fig. 5-3). Below the mucogingival junction area is the alveolar mucosa (nonkeratinized), which is continuous with the lips, cheeks, and floor of the mouth.

The marginal gingiva is made up of the gingival sulcus and the free gingival margin. The marginal gingiva in children is more rolled, flaccid, and retractable than in the adult. The child has thinner, less keratinized, more vascular gingiva, which appears redder. The orange-peel appearance of healthy adult gingiva is only seen in

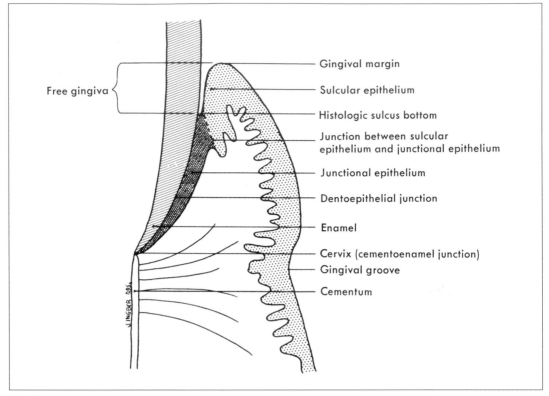

Fig. 5-1 Adult relationship of marginal gingiva to CEJ (From Goldman H M, Cohen D W. *Periodontal Therapy.* 6th ed. St. Louis: C.V. Mosby Co; 1980.)

about 35% of children.[2] Sulcus depth around primary teeth has been reported to be slightly deeper than on fully erupted permanent teeth and can be thicker and more rounded.

Variability in gingival width

The attached gingiva may become wider[3] as a patient ages, but this is insignificant in patients undergoing orthodontic treatment. The hard palate is entirely covered with masticatory mucosa, and the width of the gingiva on the labial aspect of the max-

illa and facially and lingually in the mandible may vary from 1 to 9 mm.[4] The least amount of gingiva is found on the facial aspect of the maxillary and mandibular first premolar areas and the lingual aspect of the mandibular incisors (Figs. 5-4 and 5-5). It should be remembered that in the mandible, the labial gingiva is wider on the incisors and narrows in the posterior area on the buccal aspect of the molars (Fig. 5-6). On the lingual the reverse is seen, where there is a narrow zone on the mandibular incisors and a wider gingival zone in the posterior molar areas.[5] The width of the attached gingiva must be sufficient to withstand functional demands

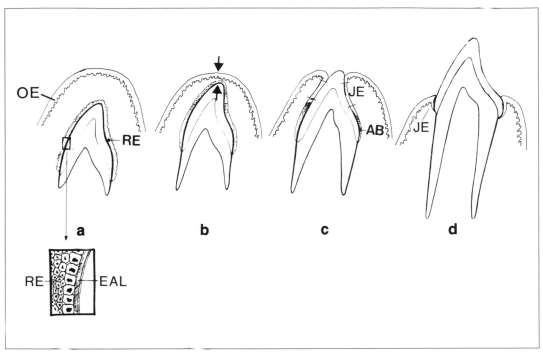

Fig. 5-2   Development of the dentogingival region with eruption of teeth. (From Lindhe J. *Textbook of Clinical Periodontology*. Copenhagen: Munksgaard; 1983.)

(a) OE-oral epithelium. Once the crown is fully formed, ameloblasts become reduced in height, produce a basal lamina, and with the outer enamel epithelium form the reduced enamel epithelium *(RE)*. Reduced enamel epithelium surrounds the crown from enamel maturation until the tooth starts to erupt. The basal lamina (epithelial attachment lamina: *EAL*) is in direct contact with the enamel and is maintained by hemidesmosomes.

(b) Once the crown approaches the oral epithelium, increased mitotic activity *(arrows)* can be seen in the outer layer of RE and the basal layer of OE.

(c) When the crown penetrates the oral epithelium, the RE and the OE fuse at the incisal edge. Apical to the incisal area, enamel is covered by a few layers of junctional epithelium *(JE)* cells. The cervical region is covered by ameloblasts *(AB)* and outer cells of the RE.

(d) During eruption, all cells of RE are transformed into junctional epithelium *(JE)*. The JE is continuous with OE and attaches the gingiva to the tooth.

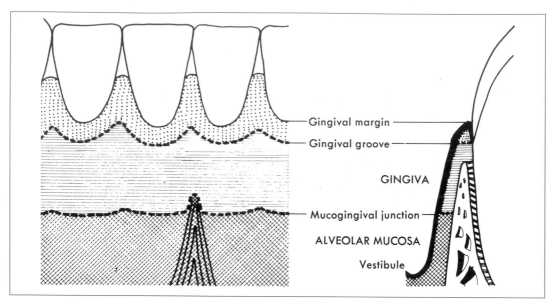

Fig. 5-3　Normal gingival relationships. (From Goldman H M, Cohen D W. *Periodontal Therapy.* 6th ed. St. Louis: C. V. Mosby Co; 1980.)

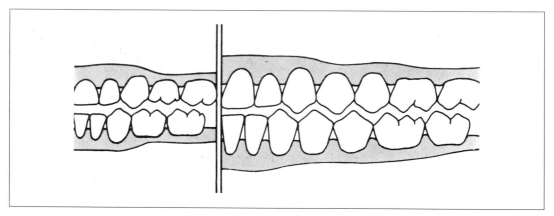

Fig. 5-4　Width of attached gingiva in primary *(left)* and permanent *(right)* teeth. (From Ainamo J, Löe H. *J Periodontol* 1966; 37:5.) "Anatomical characteristics of gingiva. A clinical and microscopic study of the free and attached gingiva" *J Periodontol* 1966; 37:5–13.

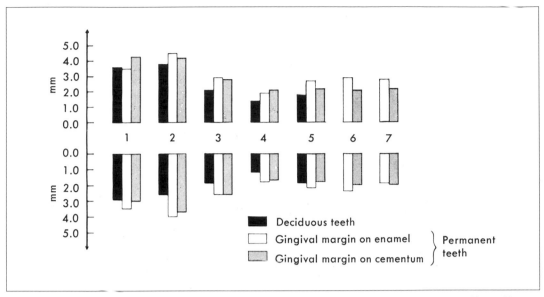

Fig. 5-5   Mean width (in millimeters) of attached gingiva in primary and permanent dentitions. (From Ainamo J, Löe H. *J Periodontol* 1966; 37:5.)

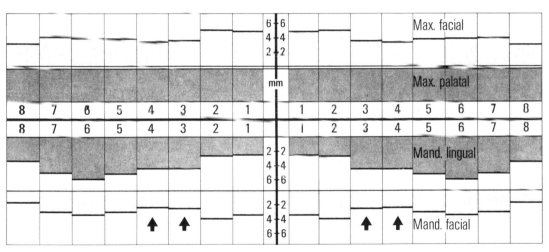

Fig. 5-6   Facial aspect of maxilla. The gingiva is wide over the incisors but narrower over canines and premolars. Palatal aspect of maxilla: the free gingival margin blends directly into the palatal mucosa without any transition zone. Lingual aspect of mandible: the gingiva is narrow in the anterior area and wider in posterior segments. Facial aspect of mandible: the gingiva around canines and first premolar is narrow *(arrows)* but wider on the lateral incisors. (From Rateitschak K H, Rateitschak E M, Wolf H F, Hassell T M. *Color Atlas of Periodontology.* New York: Thieme Inc, 1985.)

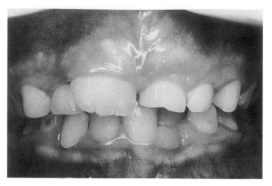

Fig. 5-7a In early transitional dentition, observe keratinized tissue over erupting permanent right central incisor and the keratinized tissue in the cervical area of the fractured primary left central incisor.

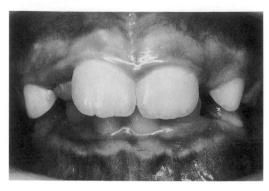

Fig. 5-7b With removal of the maxillary left primary central incisor, note inflammation of tissue over the erupting left permanent central incisor in the same area 7 months later.

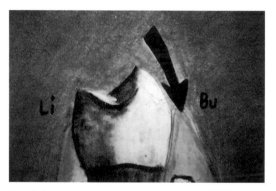

Fig. 5-8a Early stage of eruption. Note inflamed gingival margin with tissue in the occlusal one half of the crown. No protection is provided by coronal contours.

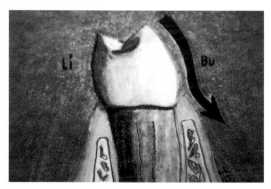

Fig. 5-8b Once the tissue has assured a more normal position on the cervical third of the crown it will show clinical health.

and maintain the integrity of the attachment during dental therapy and therefore cannot be given a minimum millimetric value.

Though sulcular depth has been reported to be greater around primary teeth than permanent,[6] the depth is greatest on erupting permanent teeth. The early adolescent (12 to 15) exhibits a "rolled," marginal gingiva because of its location in the occlusal one third to one half of the anatomic crown. Earlier during the transitional dentition (6 to 12 years), with eruption of the permanent teeth, the gingiva is attached to the incisal or occlusal portion of the permanent tooth (Figs. 5-7a and b). Tissue located above the cervical height of contours favors accumulation, retention, and growth of subgingival bacteria (Figs. 5-8a and b). During eruption of the permanent teeth, it is not uncommon to see depth of the gingival cuff up to 6 to 7 mm, particularly in the incisor area.[7]

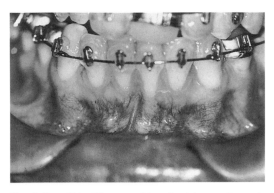

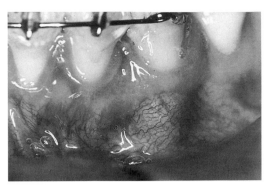

Fig. 5-9a   This 28-year-old patient has extremely thin (labiolingually) and friable tissue in the mandibular anterior area.

Fig. 5-9b   Closer view of thin tissue on left incisors and canine area.

Gingival thickness

A critical assessment must be made regarding the labiolingual thickness of the gingival tissue characteristic for a patient throughout both the maxillary and mandibular arches (Figs. 5-9a and b). Very delicate thin tissue (0.3 to 0.4 mm in thickness) as opposed to normal (0.5 to 0.8 mm in thickness) or thick (greater than 1 mm in the labiolingual dimension) is more likely to exhibit recession during orthodontic treatment. With increased gingivitis the inflammatory infiltrate spreads, the junctional epithelium is apparently disintegrated, and collagen loss occurs. The histopathology helps explain why the thin tissue type clinically responds more adversely to mild inflammatory insult, exhibiting redness, swelling, frequently spontaneous bleeding, and recession. Tooth position will influence bony topography and position of the gingival margins. Teeth in lingual version have more occlusal gingival margin, and teeth in labial position exhibit more apical gingival margin. The height and thickness of the supporting bone will also affect the position of the gingival margins, as seen in the cases of altered passive eruption described below. The patient with a thin, friable tissue type must establish exemplary oral hygiene measures before appliance placement. Inflammation must be resolved, appropriate mechanotherapy utilized, and bonded appliances used to help prevent adverse periodontal response to tooth movement.

Passive eruption

As the permanent teeth erupt into occlusion and the gingiva covers two thirds of the anatomic crown, the apical migration of the dentogingival junction (increased exposure of the anatomic crown) that follows has been termed *passive eruption*.[8] This process, allowing the crown to become fully uncovered, can take 8 to 9 years, usually stabilizing around the age of 16 years.[9] Clinical observations of the dentogingival junction in children during the transitional dentition demonstrate

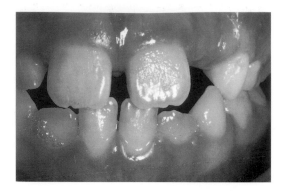

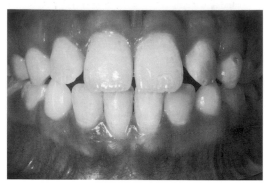

Fig. 5-10a   The transitional dentition of a patient at age 7 as permanent incisors erupt.

Fig. 5-10b   Two years later (patient is 9). Note increase in size of the clinical crown on the maxillary and mandibular incisors.

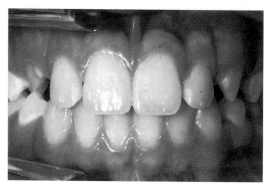

Fig. 5-10c   Same patient at 11 years of age. Continued exposure of mandibular incisor clinical crown height.

that the gingival margin is located at various heights on the anatomic crown (Figs. 5-10a to c). In adult patients the condition where the gingival margin fails to recede during tooth eruption to a level apical to the cervical convexity of the tooth crown has been described as altered (retarded) passive eruption. This condition has been called *delayed passive eruption* and is said to occur in 12 % of patients.[10] The normal alveolar crest — CEJ distance of 1.5 mm reported for adult patients is usually not seen in delayed passive eruption, and pseudopockets and lack of gingival tonus are associated with gingival tissue high on the anatomic crown.[11] In children and adolescents, however, most frequently the alveolar crest is located at the CEJ area (Figs. 5-11a to c). Although the alveolar crest is found apical to the CEJ in some patients, rarely is the alveolar crest — CEJ distance in children the 1.5 mm distance described for normal adults. Therefore, it appears that during different stages of eruption the alveolar crest — CEJ distance remains extremely small or nonexistent (Figs. 5-12a and b). A full discussion of diagnosis and classification of delayed passive eruption for adults has been reported.[11]

Gingival fiber groups

The connective tissue fiber group includes collagen, reticular, oxytalin, and elastic fibers, of which the collagen fibers predomi-

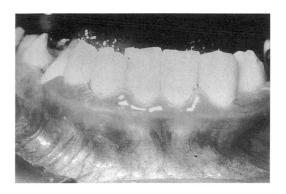

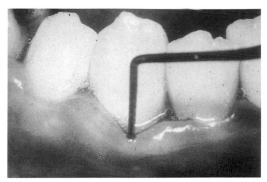

Fig. 5-11a   A 10-year-old patient has edematous, chronically inflamed gingival tissue in the mandibular anterior area.

Fig. 5-11b   Probe in place to show depth of the gingival pocket. Tissue was retractable.

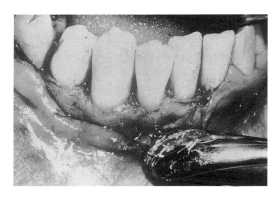

Fig. 5-11c   Bone located at the CEJ.

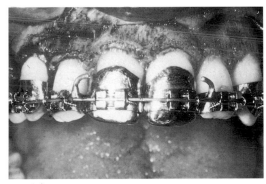

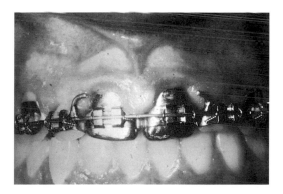

Fig. 5-12a   Gingival hyperplasia developed in the maxillary area during orthodontic therapy for this 16-year-old patient.

Fig. 5-12b   Upon gingival reflection, note that the bone is located at the CEJ on all maxillary anterior teeth.

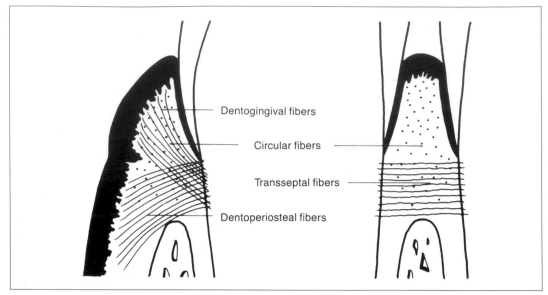

Fig. 5-13   Fiber arrangements of gingival connective tissue (From Goldman H M, Cohen D W. *Periodontal Therapy*. 6th ed. St. Louis: C. V. Mosby Co; 1980.)

nate. The collagen fibers, although randomly distributed in the tissue, have certain groups of bundles that have been divided into four groups according to their insertion and direction within the tissue: circular, dentogingival, dentoperiosteal and transseptal fibers (Fig. 5-13). These groups of collagen bundles provide resilience and tone to the gingiva, which helps maintain its architectural form. The supraalveolar and gingival crest fiber groups have been shown to be important in causing orthodontic relapse and affect postorthodontic stability.[12]

Blood supply

The main blood supply to the free gingiva is provided by supraperiosteal anastomose with blood vessels from the alveolar bone and periodontal ligament (Figs. 5-14a and b). Vessels in the coronal position of the periodontal ligament course in an occlusal direction into the free gingiva. Therefore, the free gingiva receives its blood supply from the supraperiosteal, periodontal ligament, and alveolar blood vessels.

Summary

This brief description of specific aspects of the periodontal tissues is critical for recognition of the morphologic and developmental changes seen in the periodontium of the primary, transitional, and adult dentitions. Obviously a thorough knowledge of periodontal anatomy is critical to diagnosis and for performing minor surgical procedures. Prior knowledge of periodontal anatomy is assumed, and a more comprehen-

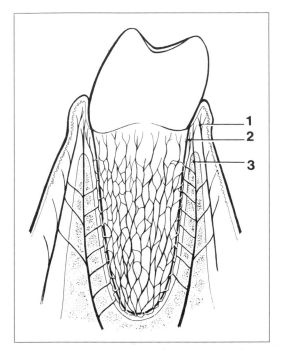

Fig. 5-14a   Blood supply to the periodontium with vessels to the free gingiva from *(1)* the supraperiosteal ligament, *(2)* periodontal ligament, and *(3)* alveolar bone blood vessels. (From Lindho J. *Textbook of Clinical Periodontology.* Copenhagen: Munksgaard; 1983.)

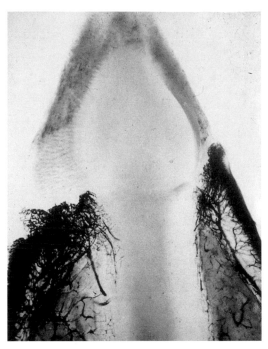

Fig. 5-14b   Note blood supply to marginal gingiva in monkey perfused with india ink. (Courtesy of D. W. Cohen, Philadelphia, Pa.)

sive review of the normal and the diseased periodontium of the child, adolescent and adult may be reviewed in current texts on pediatric dentistry and periodontics.

References

1. *Skougaard M R.* Turnover of the gingival epithelium in marmosets. *Acta Odont Scand* 1965; 23:623.
2. *Soni N N, Silberkweit M, Hayes R L.* Histological characteristics of stippling in children. *J Periodontol* 1963; 34:427.
3. *Ainamo A, Talari A.* The increase with age of the width of attached gingiva. *J Periodont Res* 1976; 11:182–196.
4. *Bowers G M.* A study of the width of attached gingiva. *J Periodontol* 1963; 34:201.
5. *Voigt J P, Goran M L, Fleischer R M.* The width of lingual mandibular attached gingiva. *J Periodontol* 1978; 49:77.
6. *Chawla H S.* Clinical evaluation of depth of gingival sulcus on primary teeth. *J Ind Dent Assoc* 1973; 45:175.
7. *Kopczyk R A, Lenox J A.* Periodontal health and disease in children: examination and diagnosis. *Dent Clin North Am* 1973; 17:27.
8. *Gottlieb B, Orban B.* Active and passive eruption of the teeth. *J Dent Res* 1933; 13:214.
9. *Volchansky A, Cleaton-Jones P.* The position of the gingival margin as expressed by clinical crown height in children age 6–16 years. *J Dent* 1975; 4:116–122.

10. *Volchansky A, Cleaton-Jones P.* Delayed passive eruption — a predisposing factor to Vincents Infection. *J Dent Assoc S Africa* 1974; 29:291–294.

11. *Coslet J G, Vanarsdall R L, Weisgold A.* Diagnosis and classification of delayed passive eruption of the dentogingival junction in the adult. *Alpha Omegan* 1977; 10:24–28.

12. *Vanarsdall R L, Musich D:* Adult orthodontic: diagnosis and treatment. In: Graber T M, Swain B F (eds): *Orthodontics: Current principles and techniques.* St. Louis: C.V. Mosby Co; 1985.

Chapter 6

Orthodontic/Periodontal Considerations for Minor Periodontal Surgery

Robert L. Vanarsdall

This chapter will highlight several types of minor periodontal surgery procedures that can prevent or correct periodontal problems, expedite treatment, reduce relapse, add to postorthodontic stability, and improve dental esthetics for orthodontic patients. Certain types of gingival morphology predispose areas to plaque accumulation and tooth decalcification (Figs. 6-1a and b). This is especially true with gingival hyperplasia, cases of altered passive eruption, and patients with acidic saliva. Zachrisson[1] has stated that gingival irritation is inevitable during orthodontic therapy whether bands or bonded brackets have been used. Marked gingival hyperplasia has been observed by all clinicans, especially for patients with poor oral physiotherapy. Coronally positioned gingival tissue tends to collect bacteria. Thickened raised tissue, with bulbous interdental papillae prevents not only self-cleaning aspects but proper oral hygiene procedures. When fibrotic, hyperplastic tissue is excised, the inflamed and damaged diseased tissue is removed and healthy tissue remains to reestablish the dentogingival junction.

In addition to the obvious improvement in gingival morphology and periodontal health, excision of gingival tissue, or gingi-

vectomy, enhances posttreatment stability.[2] Reitan[3] initially reported stretched and displaced gingival fiber bundles in dogs 231 days after rotation of maxillary lateral incisors. Later Edwards[4] reported the potential for fiberotomy to reduce rotational relapse for orthodontic patients. Moreover, parents and patients appreciate the improved dental esthetics when gingival tissue is removed from the anatomic crown of the anterior teeth.[5]

Mucogingival and soft tissue considerations

Thin tissue

In the presence of congenitally thin bone and thin soft tissue, recession can occur very rapidly. If there is a minimal zone of attached gingiva or thin tissue, particularly in the mandibular anterior area or on future abutment teeth, a free gingival graft changing the type of tissue on the tooth will help control inflammation and should be performed *before* orthodontic tooth movement begins. Thin soft tissue is not always found with thin labiolingual osseous sup-

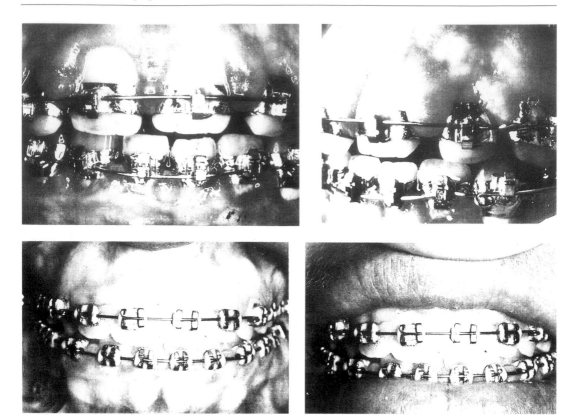

Fig. 6-1a   (upper row) Enlarged gingival tissue harbors dentobacterial plaque, and the increased pseudo-pocket depth acts as a reservoir for retention of subgingival plaque.

Fig. 6-1b   (lower row) Adolescent patient with short upper lip. Swollen edematous gingival tissues as a result of exaggerated response to mouth breathing.

port. All combinations are seen, such as thick soft tissue with a thin labial plate of bone. Little can be done to change the osseous thickness (especially the thin type) that is characteristic for the individual patient, but it is not difficult or traumatic to improve the soft tissue with a prophylactic free gingival graft.

The decision to perform preventive periodontal procedures must be made with consideration for growth and development, tooth position, type and direction of anticipated tooth movement, oral hygiene, integrity of the mucogingival junction, tissue type, inflammation, muscle pull, frenum attachment, mucogingival and osseous defects, anticipated tissue changes, and profile demands. It is always easier to prevent recession than to correct root exposure with irreversible loss of bone.

Free gingival graft technique

The recipient connective tissue bed is prepared by making an incision at the mucogingival junction extending mesiodistally to cover the desired tooth or group of teeth. With thin tissue, the epithelium should be removed to the height of the interdental papillae, the marginal and the attached gingiva with a high-speed diamond and a brushing stroke. Thin tissue should not be totally removed in bed preparation, but muscle fibers must be removed. After local anesthesia is administered, the donor tissue is dissected close to the gingival margins of the posterior teeth to obtain a uniform (1-mm thickness) graft without glandular or fatty tissue, containing no palatal rugae. The donor site can be covered with amalgam squeeze cloth impregnated with cyanoacrylate to control bleeding and a periodontal dressing applied and covered with dry foil (tinfoil).

A No. 15 Bard-Parker blade is used for dissection of the graft. The graft is sutured along the incisal edge to the interdental gingiva with 5-0 resorbable suture and a P-2 opthalmic needle. No sutures are placed apically to stabilize the graft. The graft is pressed in place with moist gauze to ensure no "dead space" beneath the graft. A surgical dressing is placed for 7 days. The dressing should be changed in 1 week and replaced for 1 additional week. Postoperative discomfort can be controlled by 500-mg acetaminophen alone.

Frenectomy considerations

Mandibular midline frenum

When a frenum is associated with a mucogingival problem it most frequently relates to an inadequate zone of attached gingiva. The high frenum insertion contributes to movement of the marginal gingiva where the keratinized tissue has been lost or detached or mechanical trauma exists. This problem is most prevalent in the mandibular anterior area and can be solved by placement of a free gingival graft (Figs. 6-2a to e).

Maxillary midline frenum

It has been recommended that a frenectomy procedure be done in the maxillary midline for young children because of the belief that the midline diastema is caused by the maxillary labial frenum. Many believe that this frenum prevents mesial migration of the maxillary central incisors, and that removal should precede orthodontic therapy. Others have suggested that if the frenum is removed, the space can be orthodontically closed more easily. However, it must be remembered that a physiologic space will normally be present between the maxillary central incisors until eruption of the canines in the adolescent dentition. In addition, a frenectomy procedure may cause scar tissue, which could prevent orthodontic space closure. With extremely large diastemata (6 to 8 mm) in the early transitional dentition, a frenectomy is usually recommended to facilitate space closure, regain space at the midline, and prevent ectopic eruption of the lateral incisors and/or canines (Figs. 6-3a and b). These interceptive early treatment problems require complete orthodontic supervision, usually additional mechanotherapy, and several stages of treatment.

A u-shaped or v-shaped radiographic appearance of the interproximal bone between the maxillary central incisors is a diagnostic key to the persistent midline diastema (Figs. 6-4a and b). This radiographic picture of the mature midline su-

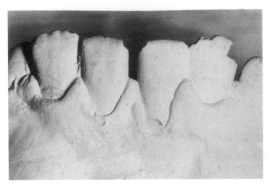

Fig. 6-2a   On the study model, observe the height of the labial gingiva on the central incisors.

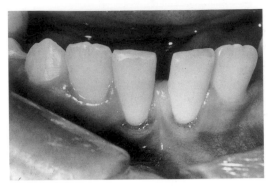

Fig. 6-2b   Several months later, note the continued gingival recession and marginal gingivitis on the facial of central incisors. Tension on the alveolar mucosa and lip will cause retraction of the gingival margin.

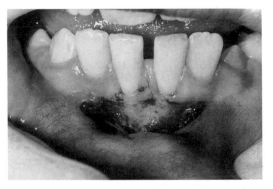

Fig. 6-2c   To prevent further recession and to create an adequate zone of gingiva, a receptor bed is prepared, leaving connective tissue and periosteum.

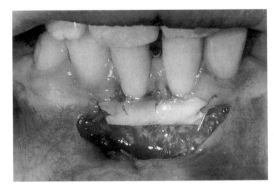

Fig. 6-2d   Donor tissue from the palate is sutured interproximally.

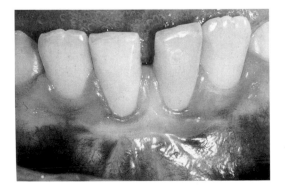

Fig. 6-2e   Postoperative result months later demonstrates no further recession and improved gingival health, even without improvement in the adolescent's home hygiene care.

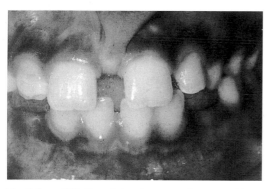

Fig. 6-3a With 7 or 8 mm between the central incisors, early removal of the frenum will allow the central incisors to move toward the midline.

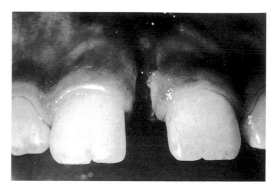

Fig. 6-3b Removal of the frenum as a space-gaining technique to allow for proper eruption of canines.

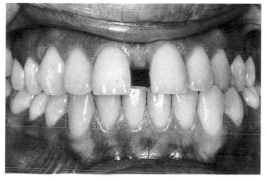

Fig. 6-4a Clinical appearance of a persistent midline diastema.

Fig. 6-4b Preorthodontic radiographic view of midline interdental bone showing v-shaped suture, which is the diagnostic key to potential relapse.

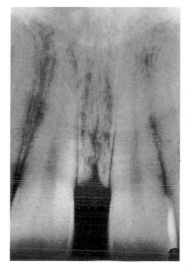

ture with firm teeth preorthodontically is indicative of relapse following excellent orthodontic treatment (no occlusal discrepancies, muscular habits or problems, tooth size discrepancies and ideal axial inclinations, overbite, and overjet.) The patient should be informed before orthodontic treatment of the need of indefinite retention with bonding of the central incisors posttreatment to prevent return of the maxillary midline diastema.

Generally, surgical removal of a maxillary labial frenum should be delayed until after orthodontic treatment, unless the tissue prevents space closure or becomes painful and traumatized. Removal may be indicated following treatment to change irreversible hyperplastic tissue to normal gingival form and to enhance posttreatment stability.

Surgical procedure

A frenectomy procedure involves excision of the entire frenum, including its attachment to bone, and removal of interdental tissue along with the incisal papilla (in the case of the maxillary labial frenum). A common complaint has been that total excision of the interdental papilla between the central incisors prevents full regeneration of the incisal papilla and can cause an unesthetic result. The proper technique to prevent this problem was presented by Corn[6] in 1964.

After administration of local anesthesia, two parallel incisions are made from the tip of the incisal papilla palatally through the center of the interdental papilla, leaving tissue on the mesial aspect of both central incisors. The incisions are carried apically to the alveolar bone, and the entire frenum and incisal papilla are removed with the exception of tissue mesial to each central incisor. The labial alveolar mucosa can be undermined by dissection to free tissue so that the wound can be sutured closed with 5-0 gut suture to prevent bleeding. The area is then covered with a periodontal dressing for one week.

Gingival retention and esthetic considerations

Mild gingival hyperplasia with orthodontic appliances seems to be transient,[7] and there is little permanent damage to the periodontal tissues.[8] Usually this condition will resolve itself or will respond to plaque removal and/or curettage. Should the gingival tissue or enlargement interfere with tooth movement, however, it must be surgically removed. Otherwise, it is preferable to wait until appliances are removed to correct abnormal gingival form with surgery.[9]

Mouth breathing

A significant problem in the orthodontic patient is the added periodontal insult of mouth breathing. The drying effect on the exposed tissue in the susceptible patient is associated with enlarged, erythematous labial gingiva, particularly in the maxillary and mandibular anterior regions. With a short upper lip, a demarcation line can usually be seen where the lip contacts the labial tissue (Figs. 6-1a and b). The mouth breather will usually exhibit dry, cracked lips as well. Though orthodontic retraction of anterior segments may help to provide a better lip seal, extraoral appliances, lip bumpers, etc, will exacerbate the problem or may even cause mouth breathing in the normal patient. The patient that exhibits symptoms of inability to breathe properly (tongue posture; enlarged adenoid tissue; narrow, high palatal vault; allergies) should be referred for evaluation of nasal obstruction and adenoid tissue. Although the plaque index is not significantly higher in mouth breathers, it has been reported that there is an increase in gingival index.[10] This increased inflammation should be reduced to a minimum before bonded appliances are placed. This is usually accomplished by scaling and curettage.

Gingiva hyperplasia

Frequently tissue will show an exaggerated response to local factors, and gingival reflection with internal bevel incision (gingivectomy) can be done to promote

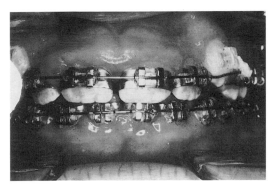

Fig. 6-5a Hyperplastic gingival tissue in adolescent girl during orthodontic treatment in the presence of mouth breathing and poor oral hygiene.

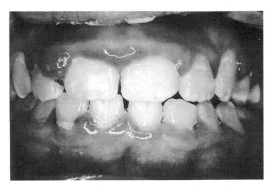

Fig. 6-5b Upon removal of orthodontic appliances, scaling and curettage are performed to reduce inflammation.

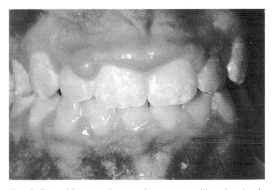

Fig. 6-5c After scaling and curettage, fibrotic gingival enlargement remains. An internal bevel gingivectomy is performed in the maxillary anterior area because of the patient's mouth breathing.

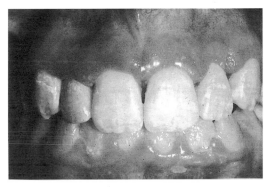

Fig 6-5d One week postoperatively, the patient has more physiologic gingival form and better dental esthetics.

stability as well as optimum esthetics and gingival topography (Figs. 6-5a to d). In adults with altered passive eruption, the gingival tissue fails to recede and the patient feels that his teeth are "short" (Figs. 6-6a and b). Many patients have thick buccal alveolar bone that must be thinned by minor osteoplasty, and if necessary a normal 1.5 mm relationship between the osseous crest and the CEJ should be established. This will prevent the return of the tissue incisally onto the anatomic crown during healing.

Contraindications

Internal bevel gingivectomy and gingival reflection procedures should not be done on the labial aspect of anterior teeth that have thin gingival tissue. Also, tissue on bell-shaped anterior teeth should only be

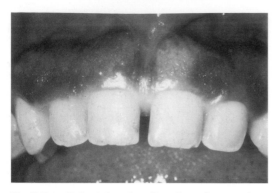

Fig. 6-6a   Patient showing altered passive eruption. During eruption, gingival margins have failed to recede to the cervical convexity of the crowns.

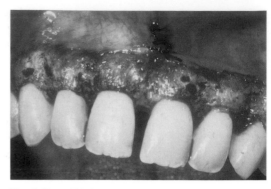

Fig. 6-6b   With bone at a normal relationship to the CEJs, the tissue is resected at a 45-degree angulation or bevel and gingivoplasty is accomplished with a diamond bur to establish ideal architecture. Patient did not desire orthodontic treatment.

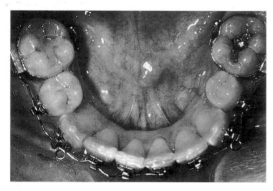

Fig. 6-7a   Mild overcorrections have been placed in the mandibular incisors.

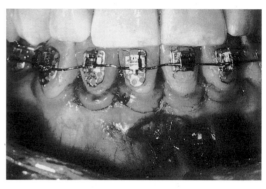

Fig. 6-7b   Sounding-type incisions are made through the incisal papilla down to bone and angled toward the tooth. The interproximal incisions are joined labially in an attempt to sound out the osseous crest. It is helpful to establish bleeding points by probing sulcular depth and marking the crestal area facially. In this case, the mandibular frenum (frenotomy) was released so that the tissue would not be retracted on the labial aspect of the central incisors.

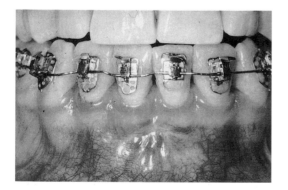

Fig. 6-7c   Two weeks postoperatively, overcorrections will be removed.

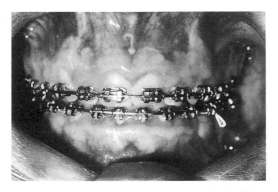

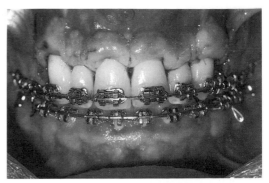

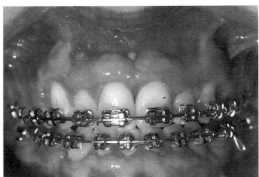

Fig. 6-8a   Gingival tissues cover two thirds of the anatomic crown of this 15-year-old boy.

Fig. 6-8b   Before appliance removal, a scalloped inverse-beveled incision to the alveolar crest is used to remove tissue on the maxillary anterior teeth. The gingiva is apically positioned and sutured interproximally with 5-0 gut suture.

Fig. 6-8c   Postoperative healing weeks later, illustrating improved gingival form, better esthetics, and enhanced periodontal stability.

reflected on the lingual or palatal aspects. The interdental tissue in these two instances may not heal back to the level of contact points, creating an unesthetic result. Spaces below the contact points are very disturbing to the patient.

Fiberotomy [11, 12]

This procedure should be done after correction of any preorthodontically rotated teeth, especially maxillary and mandibular anterior teeth such as maxillary lateral incisors in Class II, Division 2 problems. The procedure should be done prior to debonding after mild (3° to 5°) overcorrection. The overcorrection is removed one week after the surgical procedure and before im-

pressions for retainers (Figs. 6-7a to c). Internal bevel gingivectomy or labiolingual flap reflections with interproximal sutures (Figs. 6-8a to c) enhance alignment and reduce labiolingual and vertical dental relapse. These procedures should be done before fixed appliances are removed. [5]

Considerations with ectopically positioned and unerupted teeth

Many orthodontic patients exhibit teeth that have not penetrated to oral mucosa or will not erupt. Certain teeth demonstrate eruption that has been delayed significantly beyond the time when normal dental erup-

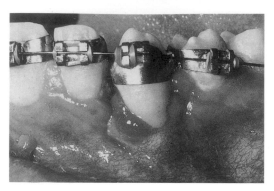

Fig. 6-9a   Adolescent patient with labial recession. Canines are typically uncovered without keratinized tissue being placed on the tooth when surgically removed.

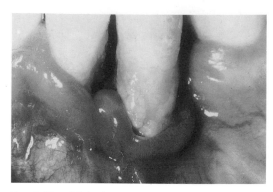

Fig. 6-9b   Clinical appearance of mandibular canine that was previously impacted and uncovered surgically.

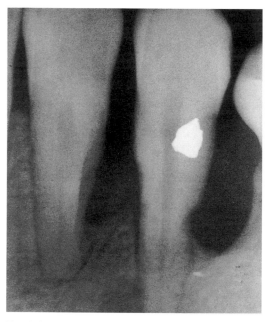

Fig. 6-9c   Radiograph of the canine showing crestal bone loss, external resorption, and devitalization.

tion for a particular patient should have occurred. Many complications (devitalization, reexposure, ankylosis, external root resorption, injury to adjacent teeth, marginal bone loss, and gingival recession) have been considered routine problems with the teeth that must be surgically uncovered during orthodontic treatment. These complications may result in prolonged treatment time, esthetic deformities, periodontal damage and, ultimately, tooth loss (Figs. 6-9a to c). With effective orthodontic and surgical management of malposed unerupted teeth, the above problems can be prevented.

Obviously, no tooth should be surgically uncovered in any fashion unless it is necessary. If a surgical procedure is required, it should be properly executed, with complete understanding of tooth development, eruption, periodontal and dentogingival anatomy, and tissue response to tooth movement. A tooth very near the occlusal plane that only has soft tissue covering can generally be rubbed vigorously by the child with an index finger; this will enable the tooth to penetrate the tissue. Conservative surgical techniques recently reported in the literature seem to lack periodontal as well as orthodontic understanding of problems with ectopically positioned teeth for orthodontic patients.[13]

Generally when a tooth has not erupted it is preferable to create space in the arch

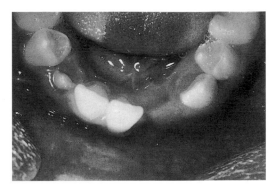

Fig. 6-10a   An 11-year-old girl in whom the mandibular left central and lateral incisors will not erupt.

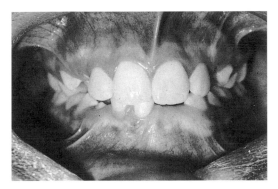

Fig. 6-10b   Occlusal view of mandibular anterior area.

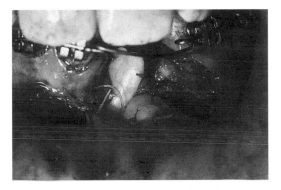

Fig. 6-10c   The mandibular arch is bonded and the archwire is placed. Individual apically positioned pedicle grafts are placed on the labial surface of each incisor.

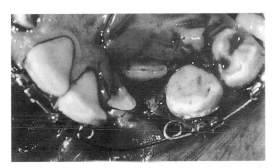

Fig. 6-10d   Occlusal view showing apically positioned pedicle grafts that were placed on the lingual aspect of each mandibular incisor. Margins of grafts are placed on the enamel coronal to the CEJ.

and allow the tooth to erupt into the arch naturally. This is possible only with teeth that are in the vicinity of the involved dental arch. Radiographs should be taken to evaluate the eruption that may or may not be occurring. If the tooth fails to erupt, stops erupting, faces away from the dental arch, or is unduly prolonging treatment time, then it should be surgically uncovered.

Once the decision has been made to uncover an ectopically positioned tooth surgically, its exact location, relative to other structures, and soft tissue management are critical.[14]

From evaluations of all necessary radiographs (cephalometric, periapical, occlusal, lateral jaw, etc), by study of the positions of the teeth in the arch, palpation, and last of all, infiltration anesthesia, it should be possible to locate the tooth precisely. It is well documented in the periodontal literature and from clinical orthodontic experience, that alveolar mucosa does not function well as a marginal tissue (Figs. 6-9a to

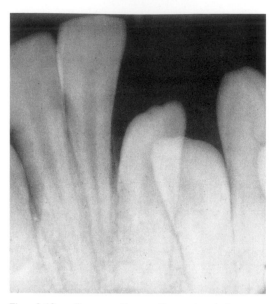

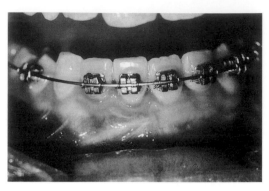

Fig. 6-10f Postorthodontic view of the incisors with grafts attached to the enamel of the left central and lateral incisors, showing normal gingival contour.

Fig. 6-10e Preoperative radiograph of the un-erupted mandibular incisors.

c). On teeth positioned labially in the maxilla and mandible, and lingually in the mandibular arch, the surgical procedure used should incorporate a means of providing attached gingiva (Figs. 6-10a to f). Mucogingival problems are avoidable provided there is proper marginal tissue placement, adequate inflammatory control, absence of excessive force, atraumatic surgery, and proper gingival attachment during tooth movement. Curettage necessary to eliminate recurring marginal inflammation should not be done overzealously (so as to impinge upon the epithelial attachment) because this may cause an apical shift of the epithelial attachment.

The cementoenamel junction area should not be distributed mechanically by instrumentation, chemically with the acid etching used for bonding, or physically by any method of attachment. This area has been pointed out as being critical with re-spect to the creation of gingival recession in animals. It is imperative, however, that most of the dental follicle material be removed so that it will not cover up the tooth or displace the graft that is positioned on the anatomic crown of the ectopically positioned tooth. It is preferred that the tooth not be bonded at the time of the surgical procedure. A dressing holds the pedicle graft against the crown of the tooth until healing (7 days) has occurred, to allow for gingival attachment.

It should be understood that not all ectopically positioned teeth can be successfully treated. However, a higher percentage of success can be achieved with unerupted teeth through attention to normal development, supporting tissue, atraumatic surgery, bonded attachments, control of gingival inflammation, and utilization of minimal orthodontic forces.

References

1. *Zachrisson B U.* Periodontal changes during orthodontic treatment. In: McNamara J A Jr, Ribbens K A (eds): *Malocclusion and the Periodontium.* Ann Arbor, Center for Human Growth and Development, The University of Michigan; 1984: 15. Craniofacial Growth Series.
2. *Boese L R. Increased Stability of Orthodontically Rotated Teeth Following Gingivectomy.* Seattle: University of Washington; 1968. Thesis.
3. *Reitan K.* Experiments of rotation of teeth and their subsequent retention. *Trans Eur Orthod Soc* 1958; 34:124–140.
4. *Edwards J G:* A study of the periodontium during orthodontic rotations of teeth. *Am J Orthod* 1968; 54:441–461.
5. *Vanarsdall R L, Musich D R:* Adult orthodontics: diagnosis and treatment. In: Graber T M, Swain B F (eds): *Orthodontics: Current Principles and Techniques.* St. Louis: The C.V. Mosby Co; 1985: chap 13.
6. *Corn H C:* Technique for repositioning the frenum in periodontal problems. *Dent Clin North Am* March, 1964.
7. *Zachrisson S, Zachrisson B U.* The gingival condition associated with orthodontic treatment. *Angle Orthod* 1972; 42:26–35.
8. *Geiger A M.* Gingival response to orthodontic treatment. In: McNamara J A Jr, Ribbens K A (eds): *Malocclusion and the Periodontium.* Ann Arbor, Center for Human Growth and Development, The University of Michigan; 1984:15. Craniofacial Growth Series.
9. *Vanarsdall R.* Periodontal considerations in corrective orthodontics. In: Clark J W (ed): *Clinical Dentistry.* vol 2. Hagerstown, Md: Harper and Row; 1978: chap 22.
10. *Jacobsen L.* Mouth breathing and gingivitis. *J Periodont Res* 1973; 8:269.
11. *Ahrens D G, Shapira Y, Kuftinec M.* An approach to rotational relapse. *Am J Orthod* 1981; 80:83.
12. *Edwards J G.* A surgical procedure to eliminate rotational relapse. *Am J Orthod* 1970; 57:35.
13. *Lundberg M, Wennstrom J L:* Development of gingiva following surgical exposure of facially positioned unerupted incisor. *J Periodontol* 1988; 59:652–655.
14. *Vanarsdall R L, Corn H:* Soft-tissue management of labially positioned unerupted teeth. *Am J Orthod* 1977; 72:53–64.

Chapter 7

The Dilemma of the Third Molar

Robert M. Ricketts

The conditions surrounding the third molars have prolonged one of the most heated and continued controversies in dentistry. In fact, the range of opinion varies from promiscuous removal and even contempt for the third molar, to an emotional bias for its preservation, to an extent beyond reason, as was promulgated by Salzman.

Many orthodontists consider the third molar a potential source of relapse. Others consider it irrelevant to mandibular anterior crowding with or without orthodontic correction.

These divergent views directly influence the different attitudes regarding diagnosis and enter into the selection of treatment modalities.

The conceived effects of the third molar also became an important aspect in polarizing clinicians toward either extraction of premolars and waiting for third molar eruption or, the opposite, expansion and arch elongation and early removal of the molar, even germectomy. Thus, the thinking regarding the consequences of the third molars may constitute a standard part of an orthodontic philosophy. Therefore, the subject is of significance to clinical actions.

Ironically, the issue of the third molar was heightened in the 1930s and 1940s, when possibilities in orthodontics were thought to be quite limited. The third molar was thought to be enlisted to help close the extraction site and to replace the function of teeth removed anteriorly. When preliminary research failed to show the thrust of the molars to be as forceful as anticipated, the champions of extraction were somewhat dismayed. At the same time, many of those choosing expansion, such as Atkinson and Brodie, were very quick to prescribe third molar removal in order to protect the stability of the enlarged arch.

It can be safely stated that the majority of clinicians would intuitively prefer to extract third molars, despite the fact that continued crowding is observed in patients in which the third molar is congenitally absent. However, general dentists are also quick to point out the difficulty of access for restorations plus the problem with hygiene. The function of third molars to many is questionable and their removal is common to the oral surgeon's training.

The controversy may have been caused by several factors, such as (1) a lack of criteria for judgment, (2) an insufficient knowledge of the method of eruption, (3) the processes of growth and space creation, (4) the performance of third molars in functional occlusion, (5) all the conditions causing crowding of the arch, and (6) the short- and long-term consequences of impaction or eruptive complications. In 1970, the author added to the dilemma by suggesting that it may be possible to identify those cases in which impaction or eruption problems could occur. Early removal or enucleation (germectomy) was also demonstrated to be safely practiced.

This chapter will deal with 12 considerations divided into four main avenues. First covered will be the lines of investigation regarding the third molars. Second, the etiology of problems and their prediction will be discussed. Third, early enucleation compared to late removal will be analyzed. Finally, indications and contraindications for third molar extraction will be covered as a basis for diagnosis and prognosis.

Investigations

The functional role of normal third molars

The first issue in the subject regards the essence of third molars. They constitute the most distal component of the trituration unit. By lying almost directly medial to the masseter muscle, they are in a position to receive a maximum crunching power.

Oberg et al in 1971, Kopp in 1972, and Bergman and Hansson in 1979 found in autopsy material and skull material a greater incidence of breakdown in subjects with loss of posterior teeth. This was consistent with the author's findings in 1967 of more radiologic disturbance with tooth loss.

The mandibular third molar normally oc-

cludes with the distal incline of the maxillary second molar together with the entire maxillary third molar. With regard to the lingual inclination of the mandibular third molar, its long axis is generally reasonably parallel to the pull of the internal pterygoid (Fig. 7-1).

Posteriorly, the occlusion interlocks horizontally and transversely, and the third molar adds to this two-dimensional stability. However, the third dimension, or the vertical, is of greater significance in that the third molar can help in the vertical support of the jaw, which helps to protect the mandibular joint from overload. In addition, by filling out the curve of Spee, the occlusion helps stabilize mandibular posture and helps keep the condyle centered sagittally. As the curve of Spee develops, the third molars make up its sharpest cant. The mandibular third molars incline mesially, while the maxillary third molars incline distally.

In a cephalometric laminographic study of 1,150 patients at a veteran's hospital from 1959 to 1969, these facts came to light. A few patients (in their 70s and 80s) with third molars well developed and in normal occlusion showed flawless joint x-rays, whereas many of those in their 20s to 40s with malocclusions or with missing teeth showed degenerative changes and joint compensations (Fig. 7-2).

Literature review

The second and third molars have been investigated by many clinical orthodontists and surgeons.[1-6] Other research investigators have made contributions, including Vego,[7] Keene,[8] Ricketts,[9, 10] and others.[11-17]

With so many studies to consider, following is a summary of the findings. Generally,

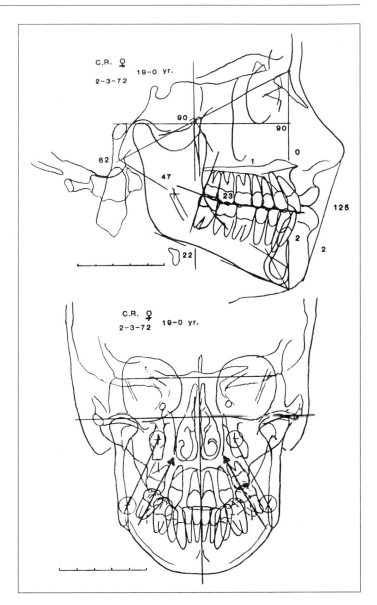

Fig. 7-1 *(A)* Lateral view shows the third molar has enough space. The manner in which the third molar fills out the curve of Spee means it is in a position to help support the vertical height to the face and to protect the condyle from overload. Note the posting of numbers for the summary analysis. *(B)* Frontal view. The long axis of the third molar *(arrows)* is almost parallel to the line of pull of the internal pterygoid muscle *(between circles)*. Due to the interlocking of the cusps, the third molar occupies a position to help stabilize the mandible from side to side.

the third molar can be a problem as an etiology of joint disease. When it supra-erupts in a Class II situation, it can cause functional interference. It is a complication to orthodontic therapy when pericoronitis develops, causing pain and tongue habits; open bite has been seen serially in such cases. The third molar is perhaps a hazard to retention in some patients. Its role in crowding is perhaps from a different mechanism than that often conceived, as will be described later.

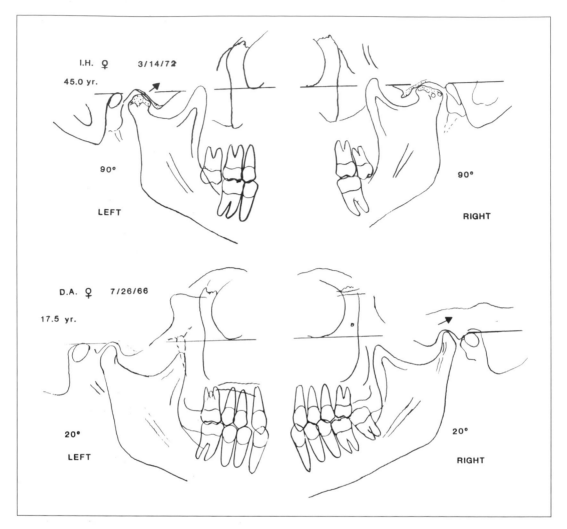

Fig. 7-2 *(A)* A 45-year-old woman with missing support in the arches, showing advanced degenerative changes with unquestionable perforation of the discs bilaterally. Notice the shortened and malformed condyles and the alteration of form with superior and anterior condyle position on the left side *(arrow)*. *(B)* A 17-year-old girl with loss of posterior support. A posterior-superior displacement *(arrow)* with flattening of the condyle posteriorly is seen on the right side with loss of first and third molars.

Early removal of the second molar frees the development of the third molar but not always with a resulting favorable occlusion. The patient may need secondary orthodontic attention to close space and finish the occlusion. If the extraction of the second molar is delayed, the mandibular third molar may never close the space from the extraction.

O'Reilly found that the removal of premolars, with forward movement of the first and second molars, did not significantly in-

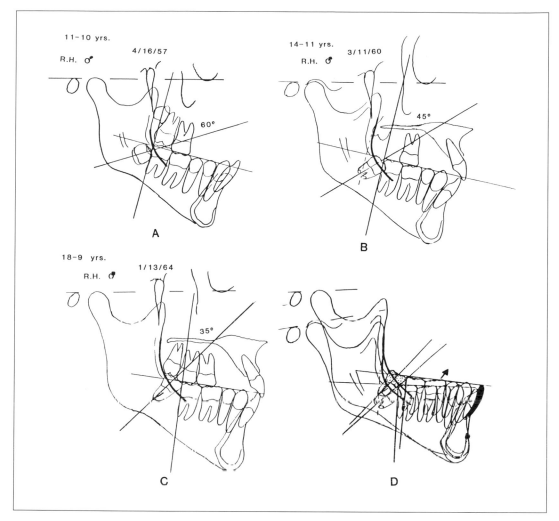

Fig. 7-3   A series of tracings showing the development of the third molar in a male patient treated with four pre-molar extractions. The buccal occlusal plane and a perpendicular line to the distal of the second molar are shown before orthodontic treatment. *(A)* The patient at age 11, showing the angle of the third molar at 60 degrees from a vertical to the occlusal plane. *(B)* After treatment, at age 14, the third molar still appears to be on its way to impaction but is angled now at 45 degrees. Note the amount of space available for the tooth at this age. *(C)* At age 18, the third molar that was badly tipped has uprighted to 35 degrees from a vertical and reached function with its antagonist. Notice 100% space for its entrance. *(D)* A superpositioning is made on the protuberance menti and on the anterior border of the ramus (which depicts the true arc of the mandible). Notice the superior and anterior eruption of the molars and the straight-upward eruption of the mandibular third molar. This is the probable modality of normal growth and explains this successful development.

crease the probability of mandibular third molar eruption or stimulate the uprighting of displaced third molar crowns, although often more space was created. In other words, the findings suggested that holding the second molar in position or pushing it backward often actually uprighted the third if it had space and was not totally trapped under the crown of the second (Fig. 7-3).

Early abortion of mandibular third molars was shown by C. Bowdler Henry in London to be practiced uneventfully in 10,000 patients. The main issue was the reliability of predicting, not the location or the technique.

About 25 % of the population has one or more congenitally absent third molars, according to the studies of Keane; however, Bjork and Palling found 16 %. It was estimated that more than one half the American population has third molars extracted. In a survey of 121 orthodontists, they reported a mean of 18 % third molars retained in nonextraction orthodontic patients.

Crowding of the mandibular arch was not contingent on the third molar's presence. A greater severity of crowding was associated with third molar presence by Keane, although when third molars were congenitally absent the molars were slightly smaller, which clouded the issue.

Predictions in children of space available by adulthood could be made to the accuracy of 90 %, which represents essentially a 1-mm error because the molar is about 10 mm wide mesiodistally. This is related to the typical and traditional viewpoint of established dentists.

Enucleation is to be recommended when the diagnosis and prognosis indicate there is insufficient space or that the third molar interferes with second molar development.

Etiology of problems and space forecasting

Third molar morphogenesis

The third molar is an extension of the primary dental lamina. The enamel is formed from ectoderm and lies dormant from birth at the retromolar trigone. Proliferation of epithelial tissue occurs at age 5. Either by the process of invagination or by the action of differential growth of bone, which has not been a consideration in the past, the embedding of the follicle starts to take place on the medial anterior wall of the ramus usually by age 7. This same characteristic was displayed for the first permanent molar before birth, and the second molar between 2 and 3 years of age or during the primary dentition's existence.

By age 8.5 years, the mixed dentition years, the follicle should be reaching mature size, and by age 9 the cap and crown state usually is present, although later development ages are observed. At age 8 or 9, the mandibular third molar crypt lies precisely in line with the buccal cusps of the teeth. Because of the narrowness of the ramus, the molar usually lies on its side and erupts with growth of the ramus, bringing its alveolus with it (Fig. 7-4).

The maxillary third molar also is a part of the original lamina and forms about midway between the base of the tuberosity and the apex of the maxillary body. It has quite an extensive distance to erupt and in fact is the last tooth to reach occlusion, often after growth is essentially completed. The maxillary third molar has been seen to erupt as much as 5 years later than the mandibular third molar (Fig. 7-5). This should be realized because the eruption of the mandibu-

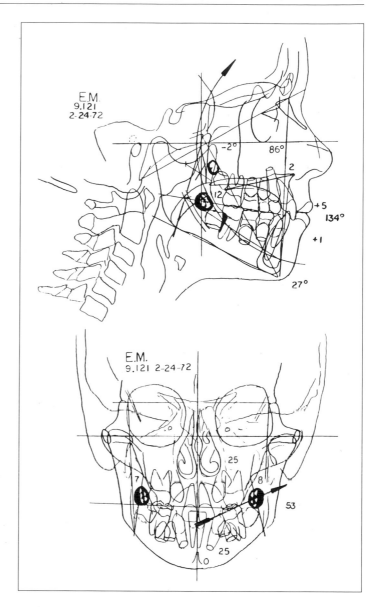

Fig. 7-4 *(A)* A 9-year-old girl showing the status of the development of the third molars. Note their location at the occlusal plane and above the second molar. Notice also the stage of formation of the maxillary third molar and its position midway between the occlusal plane and apex of the body of the maxilla above the pterygopalatine fossa. Notice that the mandibular second molar is trapped between the first molar and the third molar. Note further the space distal to the maxillary molar (12 mm) Finally note the construction of the arc for projecting mandibular growth *(arrow).* Compare to prediction in Fig. 7-14. *(B)* Frontal view. Note the position of the third molar to be inclined medially, and in a line with the buccal cusps of the occlusion in the mandibular arch *(arrow).*

lar and delay of the maxillary is often erroneously taken as an indication for extraction.

X-ray identification

While ordinary dental films have often been the sole source of diagnosis, they are perhaps the least satisfactory in yielding information regarding growth and poten-

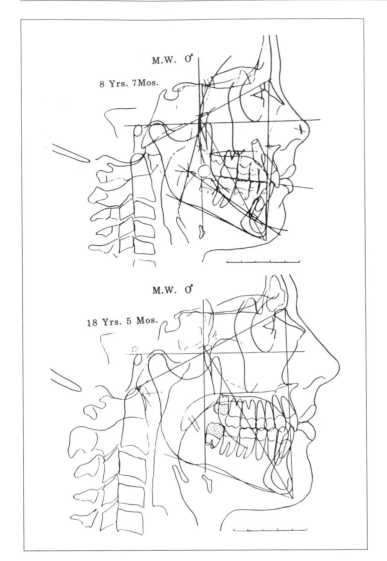

Fig. 7-5 *(A)* An 8½-year-old boy showing a normal occlusion and the position of the follicle of the third molar at the inner angle of the mandible. The patient was never treated orthodontically. Note the arc construction on the mandible. *(B)* The patient at 18½ years, showing the mandibular third molar erupted and the maxillary third molar delayed in its formation compared to the mandibular molar, which is typical.

tial impaction. This is because of their small size, the variation in angles of the central ray, intraoral film positioning, and uncertainty of the relationship to the external oblique ridge.

The panoral film is much more revealing regarding space and positioning of the third molars. While the third molars are evident and can be observed with this me-

thod, orientation in a distorted image may sometimes be questionable.

The best x-ray source for evaluation and for making projections, oddly enough, is the lateral and frontal cephalometric films. This has the advantage of standardization, reproducibility, and orientation regarding contiguous structures. In the lateral image the dentist will often be influenced by the

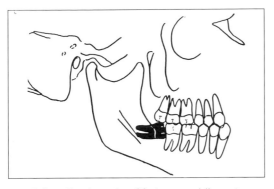

Fig. 7-6a   Tracing of a 20-degree oblique tomograph section showing an orthodontically treated patient with adequate space but a mesial angular impaction.

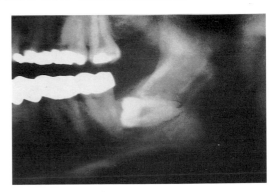

Fig. 7-6b   A woman with a horizontal impaction, showing the tip of the root in proximation with the mandibular canal. This patient likewise had adequate space for the tooth, but due to an ectopic position it failed to erupt properly.

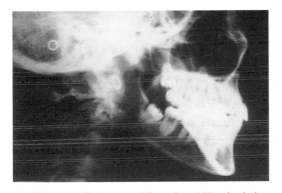

Fig. 7-7a   A 45-degree oblique head film depicting the normal development of the third molars.

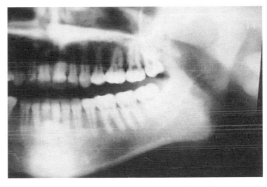

Fig. 7-7b   A panoramic film depicting the normal development of all molar teeth.

mandibular third molar relation to the external oblique ridge. In some wide mandibles the alveolar process in the human can be located lingually as the mandibular third molar erupts and functions distal to the anterior incisure of the external oblique ridge.

If tomography is available, this oriented body section method is even more revealing with regard to details in complicated cases, particularly in the 20-degree view (Figs. 7-6a and b).

The lateral jaw plate and a 20-degree to 45-degree oblique head film also are revealing, but again, this method needs study and orientation because of distortion of the image (Figs. 7-7a and b).

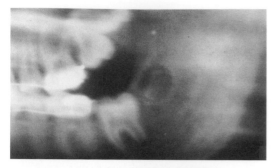

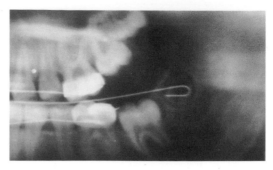

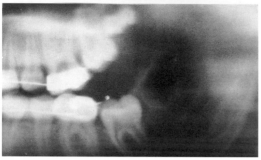

Fig. 7-8a   A patient at age 11 or 12 years, showing a late-developing third molar crypt. Note the tip of the cusps.

Fig. 7-8b   An orthodontic wire was placed along the buccal cusps and extended directly into the crypt of the tooth before its enucleation.

Fig. 7-8c   Radiograph taken at the time of surgery with the contents of the crypt removed. All radiographs were taken within a few minutes.

Developmental chronologic guides

Any definitive application or absolute dependence on tooth charts, particularly to third molars, is dangerous. Ages for formation and eruption at best can only be generalized. However, based on clinical experience, it is not uncommon to expect the mandibular third molar follicle stage to be present by age 8.5 years. Crown formation takes place on average by age 9.

The optimal enucleation time for mandibular third molars is therefore at 8 or 9 years of age. After that ime, when the crown is fully formed, extirpation of the crypt is more difficult. Larger access in the bone may be needed or the crown may need to be broken up and removed in pieces. Yet the tooth is still surprisingly high in the ramus between 10 and 12 years of age compared to its lower position later when root formation or impactions are seen. The crypt stage has been seen as late as 12 years, at which time germectomy was performed (Figs. 7-8a to c).

The maxillary third molar often is difficult to visualize because of its high position superior to the crown and, later, the roots of the maxillary second molar. Its formation lags behind that of its mandibular counterpart, as a rule (see Fig. 7-5). Its development seems to be somewhat related to space available because there are patients with eruption and root formation occurring rapidly after the second molar has been extracted and adequate space is available. It seems, therefore, more adaptive than the mandibular. Perhaps this is because of the distal inclination of the maxillary and mesial inclination of the mandibular molar.

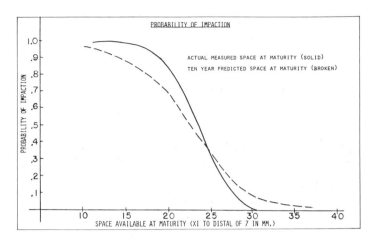

Fig. 7-9 The curves of distribution of actual measured space at maturity *(solid line)* and the predicted space in a group of patients at maturity *(broken line)*. This is the amount of space that is distal to the second molar, as measured in millimeters. Notice the agreement in the two lines with the probability in terms of percentages related to the space available.

Calculations for space required

There is a strong correlation between impaction and space available. Adequate space does not guarantee eruption, but because space is limited the chances of eruption progressively lessen (Fig. 7-9). This would suggest that methods be employed to assess the space at the junction of the ramus with the body or at the external oblique ridge, temporal crest, and trigonal area in the lateral cephalometric film.

In one technique, a plane from the second molar occlusion was extended to the external oblique ridge, and it was labeled the ramus occlusal point (RO) (Fig. 7-10). This point was useful in assessing molar position and space. Isolated cases were seen in which the third molar erupted completely behind this point, but when observed, it was even more rarely found in occlusion with the maxillary molar.

The third molar averages about 10 to 11 mm; 1 mm therefore represents about 10 % of its size. Because the third molar lies further mesially, 10 % more for each millimeter

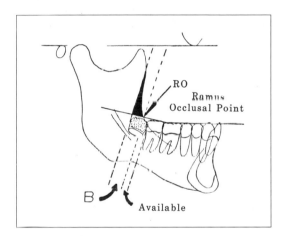

Fig. 7-10 Method of determining the point for the appraisal of space for the third molar. Lines are drawn from the distal aspect of the first molar intersecting the curve of the external oblique ridge, which is called the ramus occlusal *(RO)* point. From that point the amount of space for the mandibular third molar is assessed. Because the third molar is nearly a centimeter wide, approximately 3 mm of space is available for this tooth. *(B)* The distance behind RO; the further the tooth is behind, the poorer the prognosis.

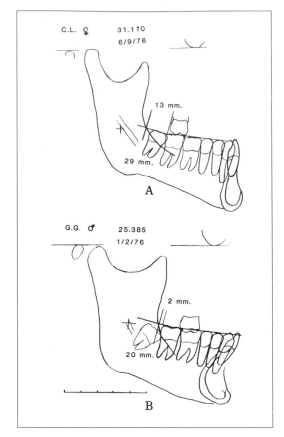

Fig. 7-11   A 31-year-old woman with a Class III occlusion showing 13 mm of space mesial to the ramus occlusal point to the distal aspect of the mandibular second molar. This is more than adequate space for the tooth. (B) The antithesis of A: a 25-year-old man, showing an impaction with only 2 mm of space available from the distal surface of the second molar to the referenced occlusal point. In A also note that the distance from point Xi to the distal surface of the second molar is 29 mm, and in B the same measurement is 20 mm. Compare these to Fig. 7-12.

of position, the chance of its eruption and function is correspondingly increased.

Thus, as a working hypothesis, if the mesial margin was found to be 5 mm ahead of point RO, the prognosis was assessed to be about 50 %. When it was 10 mm, or the full width of the molar, the prognosis was likewise at least 100 % so far as space was concerned.

This procedure has been criticized as being scientifically unsatisfactory: patients who have more than 10 mm of space would have more than a 100 % probability, which is impossible. This flaw can be addressed in two ways. One would be to make determinations from the furthest-forward second molar in occlusions in a population compared to the individual practice (with respect to racial type). For instance, third molars are seen forward of point RO in Class III — type conditions with (1) long corpus length, (2) narrow rami, (3) smaller than average teeth, and (4) generally protrusive dentures. About 13 mm is found in such extreme cases (Fig. 7-11, A).

Thus, starting with 13 mm of space rather than 10 would mean that 1.3 mm represents 10 % space. This, however, is on the side of excess, which is not the problem. Problems occur when space is limited and arch length is deficient in orthodontic patients, and when the orthodontist desires to first move molars distally or hold them in the present position for arch length problems. The assessment is critical when the molar is distal to RO.

Clinically, about 50 % of molars seem to be retained when the distal of the third molar is no more than 5 mm behind RO. One other factor is the actual size of the mandibular third molar. Smaller teeth naturally require less space.

A second consideraton, therefore, is more practical: all patients with more than 10 mm of space would not be regarded as having space problems. This would make it more feasible to consider the original idea as a working hypothesis. Thus, the farther backward the molar, the greater

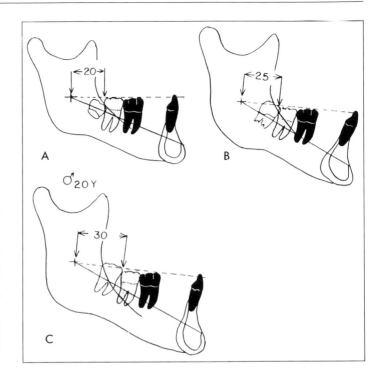

Fig. 7-12 *(A)* There was insufficient space for the third molar in this woman so it was extracted. *(B)* The more common or average relationship: the distance from the distal surface of the mandibular second molar to point Xi is 25 mm. Notice the third molar has erupted and is in position. *(C)* Note the space of 30 mm — more than enough for the developed third molar.

chance of an impaction and the less chance of eventual eruption to full function.

As protection against unwarranted removal, as projections are made, a 2-mm error is usually accepted. Therefore, among children, only those patients with 0 to 3 mm of space anterior to RO by maturity are to be considered for germectomy. In other words, when 7 to 8 mm of the tooth will be behind the anterior border, enucleation is in order.

In adults there is no question; if it is impacted, an extraction is considered. If the maxillary molar is missing or impacted, the mandibular molar may still articulate with the distal of the maxillary second molar and need not be removed. In addition, the health of the second and first molars is considered for teeth to be left as insurance.

The routine removal of all third molars on a prophylactic basis is rejected.

The opposite of excessive mandibular molar space, of course, is limited space. This is the patient with *(1)* a short corpus and square mandible, *(2)* a thick ramus, *(3)* large teeth, and *(4)* a retracted or upright mandibular denture (Fig. 7-11, *B*).

The second consideration for assessment works clinically. Other approaches may satisfy a statistician but would only complicate what is a relatively simple problem.

Another method for space evaluation was devised by Turley, who measured the space distal to the second molar from point Xi (Fig. 7-12). When the distance was only 20 mm the prognosis for third molar space was almost nil. A measure of 25 mm

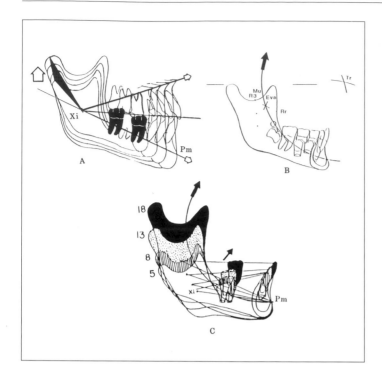

Fig. 7-13 *(A)* As noted from computer composites, the angle of the mandible bends during normal growth. From points Pm to Xi and then to condylion (at the tip of the condyle), vertical growth of the condyle takes place *(open arrow)*. The amount of bend in the mandible is 0.6 degrees per year. Notice the tendency from Xi for the anterior nasal spine and Pm to follow an allometric type shape. Note the first permanent molar gradually moves below Xi in the course of growth from 8 to 18 years. *(B)* An arc in growth was discovered from point Eva to point Pm, and that distance was used as a radius of a circle shown at the arrow. *(C)* A composite of ages 5, 8, and 13 of a serial sample of growing children, with age 18 in a sample of adult males to show normal growth on the arc. Notice the space is made for the second and third molars by the superior and anterior eruption of the mandibular teeth *(arrow)*. Little or no resorption on the anterior border of the ramus is seen.

yielded a 50 % prognosis, and 30 mm or more suggested 100 % space prognosis. Again, in this hypothesis the prognosis would change 10 % for each 1 mm of space.

Predicting available space for mandibular molars

In order to predict how much space will be available for third molars in the adult, a projection must be made of the growth of the mandible in the child. After that, the development of the occlusal plane and teeth are projected, and the behavior of the mandibular first molar, once determined, can be used as a guide for the second molar's position. From that, the third molar space can be calculated by using either points RO or Xi.

Fig. 7-13 illustrates how these calculations are made. Longitudinal computer composites show the mandible to bend at a rate of 6° per year (Fig. 7-13, *A*). Point Pm is shown by implants to be stable. A search for the true arc leads to the location of point Eva at the base of the coronoid process. The distance between points Eva and Pm is used as a radius of a circle to create the arc (Fig. 7-13, *B*). The arc is extended from the sigmoid notch at a rate of 2.5 mm per year. Variable growth behavior of the condyle is made depending upon type. The external oblique ridge is projected off the arc by adding 0.3 mm per year to the anterior border of the ramus at point Rr.

Striking predictions have been produced in untreated patients. Also, excellent results were projected for first molar behavior with known treatment modalities (Fig. 7-14).

The first molar was noted to erupt 0.5 mm per year directly vertical to the original corpus axis (only 5 mm in 10 years). It is very important to realize that the occlusal plane tends to behave with point Xi (and the mandibular first molar erupts slightly less because of the development of the curve of Spee) (Figs. 7-13, *A*, 7-14, *B*, and 7-15b). The maxillary third molar can be measured from the pterygoid vertical coordinate. This line is determined by a perpendicular to Frankfort plane at the posterior margin of the pterygopalatine fossa. It can be carried over on subsequent tracings from its crossing with the BaN line. From that reference, the maxillary molar starts at a position at 3 mm plus the patient's age (add 1 mm per each year) (Figs. 7-15a and b).

Factors in eruption

From 1771 until 1971 it was generally accepted that eruption space for the mandibular third molar was made by resorption of the anterior border of the mandible. This theory was based on the hypothesis of Hunter in 1771, a wire embedding of the pig mandible by Humphrey in 1868, and the madder-root feeding of pigs by Brash in 1928. The theory was altered by Bjork's implant studies in 1963 and further modified by the concept of arcial or spiral growth by Ricketts in 1965 and 1970 and Moss in 1970.

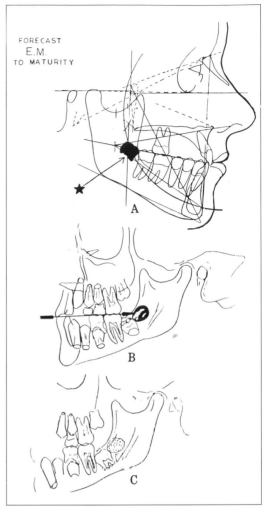

Fig. 7-14 A projection made on the girl shown at age 8 in Fig. 7-4. *(A)* Notice the prediction of inadequate space for the third molar as this patient would be corrected for malocclusion and grow to maturity. *(B)* An oblique tomogram, showing the crypt and the early calcification of the tips of the teeth at age 9. *(C)* Note the removal of the crypt and its contents.

Hundreds of successful predictions strongly suggested that the lower border of the mandibular angle resorbs and the mandible grows on a curve. It is inconsistent with nature that heavy bone would be

Fig. 7-15a   Normal growth as depicted from position 1 (the "four position analysis"). Notice the maxillary molar (from the constructed pterygoid vertical carried over from the first tracing) shows a movement forward of 1 mm each year. Notice the path of the maxillary first molar is in a general interior-anterior direction with the facial axis. As the maxillary molar moves anteriorly, space is made for the second and third molars. This normal space is usually a patient's age plus 1 mm per year.

Fig. 7-15b   Position 3, showing the gradual migration of the maxillary denture forward on the maxilla. The maxilla grows at a rate of 0.6 mm per year from the palatal plane and moves forward 0.3 mm per year from the anterior nasal spine. Notice the change in the occlusal plane as the maxillary denture follows the growth in the mandible.

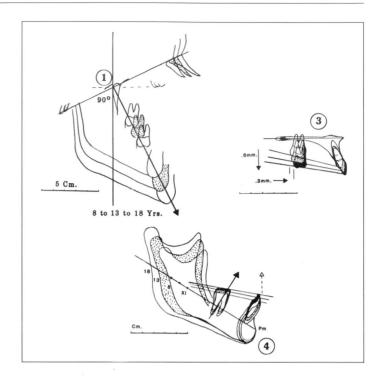

Fig. 7-15c   Position 4, showing the mandibular molar erupting at about 0.5 mm per year in a direct vertical position from the original corpus axis, (or Xi-Pm). Notice that the incisor erupts slightly more and in a superior and posterior direction to account for the leeway space from age 8 to age 13.

laid down on the external ridge only to be wasted by resorption for space for teeth. The truth is, the mandible does not resorb to any remarkable degree, and the impression of anterior ramal resorption is gained by erroneous superpositioning on the lower border of the mandible.

The arc growth forecast method shows that space is actually achieved by superior and anterior continued eruption of the whole dental arch (Fig. 7-16).

This fact is revealed by findings of first permanent molars showing early ankylosis in which the roots are fused with bone and become deeply buried in the bone. These end up near the cortical plate at the inferior margin of the corpus (Fig. 7-17).

This finding of a natural implant indicates the extensive superior and anterior eruption of the mandibular arch.

With the comprehension of arc growth and forward arch migration, it can readily be visualized how a horizontal position of the mandibular third molar can upright. Because the molar initially lies at a mesial angle and growth on the arc continues, the actual eruption is in a more vertical direction rather than just an uprighting of the entire tooth (see Figs. 7-3 and 7-13).

It is well known that loss of the mandibular first permanent molar often is accompanied by a distal drift of the second premolar, which may be followed by a deepening of the bite, and a supraeruption of the ca-

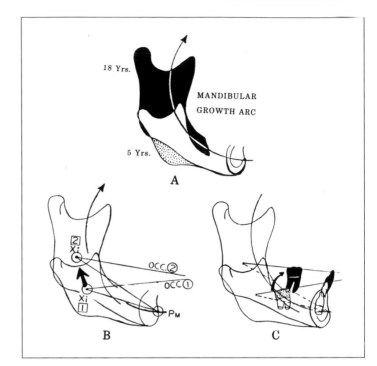

Fig. 7-16 *(A)* The mandibular growth on the arc in a male patient from ages 5 to 18 years. *(B)* Notice that during this time the occlusal plane changes with point Xi. *(C)* As the occlusal plane changes, the mandibular first permanent molar erupts superiorly and anteriorly, as does the mandibular incisor. This illustration depicts the author's concept of development of the mandible and eruption of the mandibular teeth, which is confirmed in Fig. 7-17.

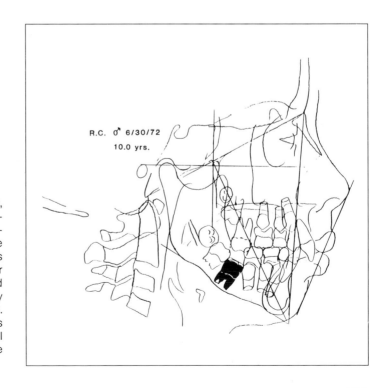

Fig. 7-17 A boy at age 10 years, with early ankylosis of the mandibular first molar. It has almost penetrated through the border of the mandible as the mandible has grown on the arc; the lower border of the mandible has not resorbed in a normal manner. The maxillary molar has erupted into the space. Mandibular molars sometimes must be removed from an external approach to the mandible. (Case courtesy of Dr R. Coulsen.)

nines. During the eruption process the molar's mesial migration is actually slowed, while the mandibular incisors continue to erupt, the lips and mouth muscles containing the anterior segment.

This would suggest that the first molar produces a mesial force component in keeping with continued eruption along the line of its strong, distally inclined distal root. The second also has a mesial inclination and action.

Miura[18] reported findings on the force of eruption of teeth in experimental animals. Small gauges were placed on the erupting incisor of a rabbit on one side, while the other side was used as a control. A force of 3 g slowed eruption, a magnitude of 5 g stopped it, and 7 g intruded it. Further studies suggested that optimum tooth movement occurred at about 0.8 g/mm^2 of enface root surface. These studies showed that an eruptive force did exist.

In a separate clinical study, meanwhile, Ricketts, after consultation with Dr B. Lee, had arrived at a desirable 1.0 g/mm^2 per square millimeter for enface root movement. Calculations of blood pressure and surface areas suggested the hypothesis that about 0.2 g/mm^2 was probably active in the eruptive stage.

Because the enface of the molar roots are 50 to 80 mm^2, the potential eruption force would be 50 x 0.2 g = 10.0 g, or 80 x 0.2 g = 16.0 g. Because this force is more in line with the contact areas of the mandibular teeth, as the third molar is erupting, this 12 to 16 g of force could possibly be a small factor in jamming of the arch, in addition to other factors such as conditions of tight lips or closed bite. This mesial component is particularly effective when added to the first and second molars, which may have the same potential or another 24 to 32 g,

making a total of about 40 g, or nearly 1.5 oz, during the whole developmental period.

With regard to crowding potential in the mandibular arch, three other facts should be remembered. First, the first and second mandibular molars also contain this eruptive drive. The third merely adds to those rather than being an independent factor. Also, all impactions are not of the same type as assumed by virtually all studies regarding their effect on the mandibular arch from the posterior. Some patients have molars erupting distally. Calculation of only the distal roots, which are inclined anteriorly, would yield estimates of as low as 16 g for the combined first and second molars, with 8 g more, or 24 g total, when all three are present (Figs. 7-18a and b).

The second factor is the consideration of events at the anterior end of the arch. As the incisors on the arc erupt superiorly and anteriorly, the arches are contained by the lips (see Figs. 7-13 and 7-16). In normal and deep bite conditions, the lower lip embraces the maxillary incisors and in turn holds the mandibular. In deep bite with maxillary protrusion and in open bites, the lower lip alone acts as a stop to the anterior migration. Thus, a tight lip can cause crowding by containing the denture anteriorly, while eruption force is active posteriorly to produce a jam in the arch (Fig. 7-19).

The third factor in crowding is the inclination of incisors and canines and the conditions of the bite. Vertical angles or interincisal angles above 130° theoretically put more force on the mandibular anterior teeth because of the lingual incline of the maxillary incisor. With clenching and bite settling, the teeth may become crowded and relapse more severely.

The foregoing conditions are occa-

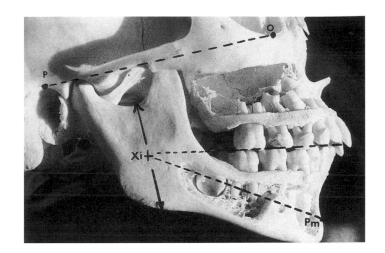

Fig. 7-18a   The position of the occlusal plane in a mixed dentition skull and the position of the second molar faced inward in its position at approximately age 8. Notice the occlusal plane is almost exactly on point Xi.

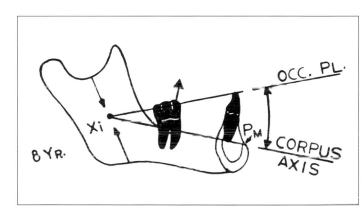

Fig. 7-18b   The angle between the corpus axis and occlusal plane tends to be orderly in natural development.

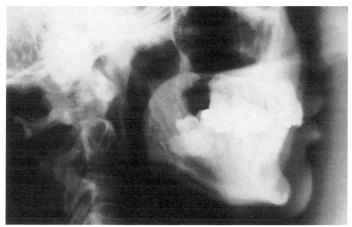

Fig. 7-19   An adult with a tight lower lip and asymmetry in the mandible, showing a distal angular impaction on one side and a mesial angular impaction on the opposite side.

sionally demonstrated in treated patients with a 4-to-4 (or 3-to-3) fixed retainer in place, as eruption force on the anterior segment is limited by the lower lip while the mandibular third is asserting itself. The second premolar in this event is deflected out of the line lingually. Thus, the etiology of the crowding and relapse, theoretically, can be due to a combination of molar force, anterior lip containment, vertical incisor positions, a settling of the bite, and a rebound of the mandible as age ensues — in other words, it is a multifactorial cause.

Maxillary molars

Less jamming is seen from the maxillary molars because the direction of eruption is buccal and posterior. When the maxillary first permanent molar rotates before its eruption, it too can jam the primary maxillary arch, causing erosion of the distal root of the second primary molar. It is important, therefore, to control the paths of all molar eruptions when these teeth are in undesirable initial positions. The same resorption can take place from the maxillary third molar against the roots of the second, although this is more rare.

Two further principles should be kept in mind. First, a tooth will follow a line of least resistance in its eruption. For example, distal eruption of the mandibular second molar will occur when the third molar crown or crypt is removed (Fig. 7-20). Secondly, a tooth locked into an unfavorable position may "spin its wheels," so to speak. It will eventually lose its eruptive potential and erupt very slowly when relieved of crowding.

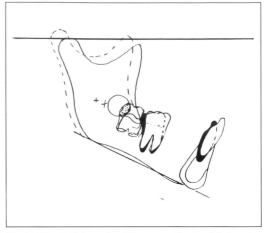

Fig. 7-20　In this patient the mandibular third molar was enucleated and a utility arch was placed, tipping the mandibular first molar posteriorly and intruding and retruding the mandibular incisors. Notice that the second molar has erupted distally to occupy a position in some of the space made by the removal of the follicle of the third molar.

Early vs late third molar removal

Surgical technique for germectomy

The third molar crypt lies precisely in line with the buccal cusps of the primary and secondary molars (Figs. 7-21a and b). For anesthesia, a mandibular block is used, and in some excitable children a small injection (0.5 ml) is placed directly in this crypt, which also helps to control bleeding. In addition, a long buccal branch block is performed because of possible involvement with the buccinator muscle.

After the external oblique ridge (Fig. 7-22a) is located, a straight scalpel or electrosurgical unit is used to make an in-

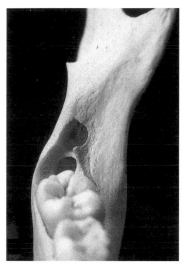

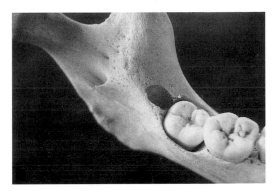

Fig. 7-21a   A developing mandible in a child, showing the position of the crypt directly in line with the buccal cusps. The pit immediately behind the mandibular first molar is the development of the third molar.

Fig. 7-21b   An internal view of a dried mandible specimen. Notice the position of the third molar crypt above and behind the developing second molar. Note further (at the triangular plane below the sigmoid notch) the number of vascular channels on the medial aspect of the ramus, which is actually its tuberosity.

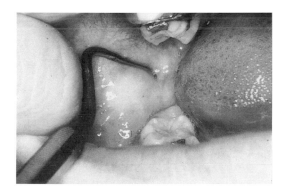

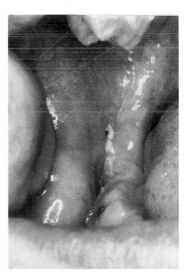

Fig. 7-22a   The inside of a mouth, locating the medial border of the external oblique ridge and palpating for the crypt for the third molar. Note that there is a slight groove or crease in the retromolar-trigone area.

Fig. 7-22b   An electrosurgical cut was made just in line with the buccal cusps.

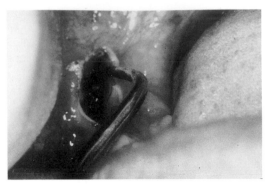

Fig. 7-23a   A spoon excavator is placed in the crypt.

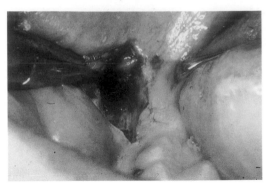

Fig. 7-23b   The contents have been removed and the hemostat is used to remove any of the Hertwig sheath.

cision of about 1 cm just at the crease or buccal connection in the mucosa distal to the first molar (Fig. 7-22b). The crypt lies buccal to the incision, but the tissue can be elevated buccally in order to prevent cutting of the muscle fibers. The opening to the crypt is exposed with the periosteal elevator, and it is located well above the second molar crown and lingual nerve (Fig. 7-23a). *Do not try to go lingually with the elevation, because the lingual nerve can be damaged.*

The contents of the crypt are removed with spoon excavators. A careful scraping of the crypt is accomplished, and any remnants of the sheath are removed with a small hemostat (Fig. 7-23b). If the opening is small, no suturing is required. Minor swelling and pain will be expected. Healing is fast and remarkably uneventful compared to impaction surgery. No dry socket has ever been encountered because no root socket is present. The contents should be the membrane, the gel-like matrix of the crown, and perhaps some cusp tips (Fig. 7-24).

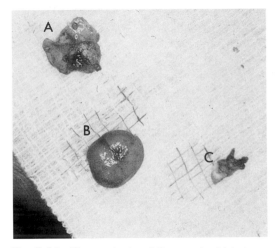

Fig. 7-24   The contents of the crypt which have been removed. *(A)* The membrane; *(B)* the follicle; *(C)* the tip of the cusps that were present.

Longitudinal study of results of early removal

Enucleated third molar patients are followed serially with regard to their behavior. My initial inexperience resulted in the caps of crowns not being removed in two patients. (The cap had formed after the last x-ray was taken.) In one the cusp-cap was later exfoliated. In the other, it remained dormant

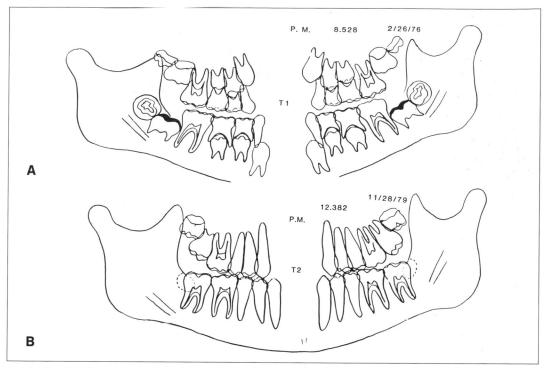

P. M.   8.528   2/26/76

T 1

A

11/28/79

12.382

P.M.

T 2

B

Fig. 7-25   (A) T1 shows tracings of panoramic right and left sides in an 8½-year-old boy, taken in 1976. The third molars were enucleated and treatment was initiated. (B) T2 age 12. The mandibular second molars have erupted distally into the space previously occupied by the third molar.

and was later easily located and removed in a minor procedure.

The overwhelming benefit, as mentioned previously, was the distal movement of the mandibular second molar into the crypt of the removed third and the freeing of the second molar to erupt optimally (Fig. 7-25).

Timely removal of the maxillary third molar at age 13 to 15 may sometimes be needed to prevent buccoversion of the maxillary second molar in patients having received orthodontic distalization of the first molar. In rare cases, the second molar is removed in order to circumvent cross-bite treatment at a later age. As mentioned before, the maxillary third molars usually erupt favorably and rapidly in that event.

Indications and contra-indications for extraction

Management of problems of the third molars

Fundamental to any treatment or diagnostic and prognostic regime is the understanding of the process of normal development and of the possible pathoses and complications (Figs. 7-26a and b and 7-27).

To reiterate, the eruption of the total mandibular arch is characterized, on the arcial expression, as being superior and anterior. When undergrowth on the arc ensues, or

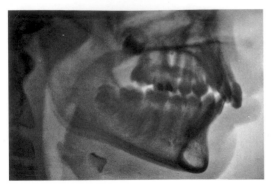
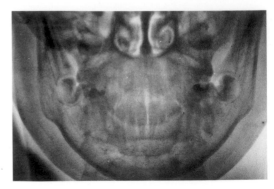

Figs. 7-26a and b   Lateral and frontal headfilms of a male patient with a follicular cyst prior to treatment, showing the position of the crypts of the third molars. Notice on the right side in the frontal view at the angle of the mandible there is a slightly enlarged crypt (on the medial side), but not enough to warrant a diagnosis of a cyst.

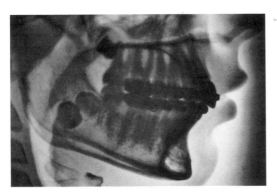
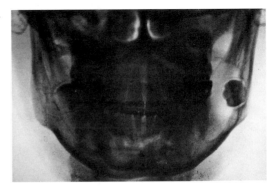

Figs. 7-26c and d   One year later. Note in the lateral view the displacement of the molar on one side down toward the angle of the mandible. Note in the frontal view the displacement of that third molar all the way to the lateral border of the ramus, with the development of a follicular cyst.

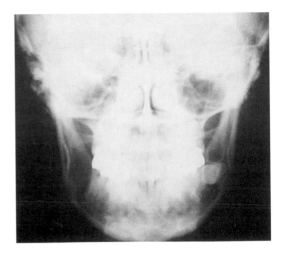

Fig. 7-27   Frontal headfilm showing an impaction of the mandibular third molar on the right side. The root tip is precisely in the mandibular canal.

Fig. 7-28 Intraoral films showing the technique for replacement of a loop with a wire spring under impacted third molars in an extraction. A second technique would be to bond a bracket onto the tooth in order to apply pressure on the tooth, but in these conditions below the soft tissue it is most difficult to maintain an attachment. Therefore, the wire is the most successful.

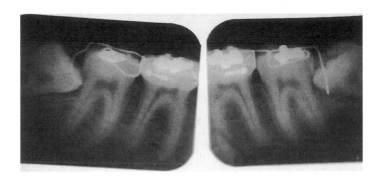

when the limiting influence of the buccinator muscle and periosteal contraction, together with the lower lip complex, inhibits anterior drift, a lack of space becomes evident. These two factors account for the etiology of mandibular third molar impaction. Ectopic position of the crypt or inclination of the crown to a horizontal or inverted position can be a third factor even when space is adequate.

When extraction of premolars is performed, the older tieback techniques with edgewise methods result in half the extraction site being closed by the molar forward movement. Because the premolar ranges around 7 mm, a 3.5 mm additional posterior space would be produced. In our analysis of space, treatment should increase the odds of space available by 35%. In contemporary bioprogressive therapy, the space lost may be none at all, or only as much as 20%. It may be necessary, therefore, in occasional cases, to further treat the third molar even in premolar extraction conditions if they are to be retained.

Options

In correcting the mandibular third molar, the second and first molars are useful. A horizontal loop with a smooth hook is placed under the unerupted crown. The wire is a reduced rectangular wire placed under the third molar crown. This technique produces a decided uprighting effect (Fig. 7-28), and local anesthesia will help in placing the wire at first.

Another procedure is to bond a bracket on the occlusal surface and place a distal-superior force on the crown to turn in backward. The tendency is to put more than enough force on the loops to do the job, displacing the anchor units. No more than 50 g of continuous force is needed to tip the tooth adequately.

Another technique for minor cases, before the maxillary molar has erupted, is a simple separation wire tie. The unlocking will stimulate favorable development.

Finally, bonding on the buccal surface can sometimes manage the molars most efficiently.

Early removal of maxillary second molars can produce even more rewarding results than can be achieved with their mandibular counterparts. Often the maxillary third molar will erupt entirely anteriorly, particularly when the second molar is removed by age 12 or 13, but sometimes it does not. The early removal of maxillary third molars frees the second molar roots to be positioned accordingly with appliances.

Use of the computer in diagnosis and prognosis

Experience suggested that three attitudes developed following the third molar movement. One was to reject the whole idea as nonsense. The second was to remove the buds when radiographs suggested any suspicious conditions. A third, and the correct viewpoint, was to routinely make long-range projections in children by the age of 8.

Projections can be made with and without orthodontic treatment in order to determine the space to be available with growth and the differences that treatment will make. Many clinicians are not prepared to produce long-range growth predictions. Even if they have learned the procedure, they do not have time to conduct such exercises on a routine clinical basis. This problem, therefore, lends itself very favorably to the computer or a commercial laboratory service. Such calculations are available from commercial enterprises. As personal in-house computers become known, the whole attitude will change.

Probability tables can be adapted. Projections concerning impaction, eruption, and eruption to full function are the three considerations. By using Baye's Theorem, a curve was derived to represent the chances of third molar eruption as a function of the distance from point Xi to the distal side of the second molar. Retesting of the programs proved accuracy to be at 90%.

Conclusions

Twelve different studies need to be covered in a logical sequence for consideration of the third molars.

The third molars support normal occlusion and the TMJ when in proper position. These teeth should be maintained unless pathologic with respect to the second molar and/or to the integrity of the jaws.

One cause of impaction is significantly related to available space. Crowding in the mandibular arch can be influenced by the third molar in more than a passive manner. Mesial drift of all molars and an anterior component in occlusal function also may be factors. However, imbrication is also caused by containment of the denture by tight lips, tension of connective tissue, deep bite, high interincisal angles, and vertical growth patterns, during the mesial migration of all the molars.

The mandibular third molar is usually, but not always, developed sufficiently to diagnose and can be removed when the patient, male or female, is 8 or 9 years of age, although the variation in calcification is great. This procedure is called enucleation, or germectomy.

Methods for predicting space availability have advanced to the stage that a probability exists for sufficient accuracy for regular clinical use. Adequate prognosis can be made for both maxillary and mandibular molars. Space is accurately revealed from the technique of the arc of growth of the mandible and, by extension, of the corpus axis and prediction of the buccal occlusal plane. Maxillary projections are calculated from the pterygoid vertical and are managed later.

With premolar extraction, one survey

suggested that two thirds of third molars were removed or absent by adulthood; less than one fifth retained third molars in nonextraction orthodontic cases.

Early surgical removal of the follicle or the developing crown is relatively innocuous and uncomplicated when compared to later impaction procedures. Training and education for the detail of its use is necessary. The tooth is located on the occlusal plane at age 9.

Early, third molar germectomy or removal (by age 12) frees the development of the second molars and is an alternative to extraction of premolars or second molars. When second molar extraction is done later than age 14 the space may not close.

Ectopic third molars can be saved when space is adequate. The patient should at least be given a choice in the matter.

The computer can help with the diagnosis and the prognosis. The best long-range estimates come from cephalometric films.

The third molar is of great concern for all of dentistry, but most of all to orthodontists in treating the developing dentition.

References

1. *Chipman M.* Second and third molars: their role in orthodontic therapy. *Am J Orthod* 1961; 47:498–520.
2. *Ledyard B C.* A study of the mandibular third molar area, *Am J Orthod* 1953; 39:366–373.
3. *Humerfelt A, Slagsvold O.* Changes in occlusion and craniofacial pattern between 11 and 25 years of age. *Trans Europ Orthod Soc* 1972; 113–122.
4. *Bergstrom K, Jensen R.* Responsibility of the third molar for secondary crowding. *Dent Abstracts* 1961; 6:544.
5. *Henry C B, Morant G M.* A preliminary study of the eruption of the third molar tooth in man based on measurements obtained from radiographs, with special reference to the problem of predicting cases of ultimate impaction of the tooth. *Biometrika* 1936; 28:378–472.
6. *Laskin D.* Evaluation of the third molar problem. *Am Dent Assoc* 1971; 82:824.
7. *Vego L.* A longitudinal study of mandibular arch perimeter. *Angle Orthod* 1962; 32:187–192.
8. *Keene A J.* Third molar agenesis, spacing and crowding of teeth and tooth size in caries-resistant naval recruits. *Am J Orthod* 1964; 6:445.
9. *Ricketts R M.* Roentgenographic study of degenerative disease of the mandibular joint. Presented at the Annual Meeting of the International Association for Dental Research, March 20, 1964, Los Angeles.
10. *Ricketts R M.* A principle of arcial growth of the mandible. *Angle Orthod* 1972; 42:368–386.
11. *Kaplan RG.* Mandibular third molars and postretention crowding. *Am J Orthod* 1974; 66:411–430.
12. *Ricketts R M, Turley P, Chaconas S, Schulhof R.* Third molar enucleation, diagnosis and technique. *J Calif Dent Assn* April 1976; vol 4 (4):52–57.
13. *Schwarze C W.* The influence of third molar germectomia — a comparative long-term study. In: Cook JT (ed): *Transactions of 3rd Int Orthod Congress.* St. Louis: C.V. Mosby Co; 1975.
14. *Richardson M E.* Late lower arch crowding: facial growth or forward drift? *Europ J Orthod* 1979; 1:219–225.
15. *Richardson M E.* Lower molar crowding in the early permanent dentition. *Angle Orthod* 1985; 55:51–57.
16. *Lindquist B, Thilander B.* Extraction of third molars in cases of anticipated crowding in the lower jaw. *Am J Orthod* 1982; 81:130–139.
17. *Bishara SE, Jakobsen JR, Stasi MJ, Treder JE.* Changes in the maxillary and mandibular tooth size — arch length relationship from early adolescence to early adulthood: longitudinal study. *Am J Orthod* 1989; 95:46–59.
18. *Miura F.* Effect of orthodontic force on blood circulation. In: Cook JT (ed): *Transactions of 3rd Int Orthod Congress.* St. Louis: C.V. Mosby Co; 1975.

Chapter 8

Orthodontic Management of Traumatized Teeth

Olle Malmgren / Barbro Malmgren

This chapter describes the influence of traumatic injuries on orthodontic treatment plans and assigns treatment principles in patients with severe traumatic injuries of the teeth. Treatment planning of patients with traumatized teeth is a complicated evaluation of both the prognosis for the injured teeth and for treatment of the malocclusion. A coordinated treatment plan is necessary before orthodontic treatment is initiated. This plan should be based on a realistic evaluation of the prognosis for the injured teeth. Accordingly, this chapter begins with a short presentation of general treatment principles for traumatized teeth. Clinical and radiographic findings of healing and complications after dental injuries are discussed before presentation of orthodontic treatment plans. For a more extensive description of general treatment principles for traumatized teeth, the reader is referred to J.O. Andreasen, *Traumatic Injuries of the Teeth*.[1]

Epidemiology

Dental injuries in the permanent dentition are most frequent between the ages of 8

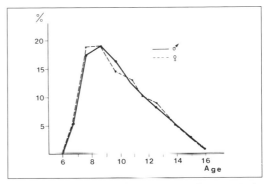

Fig. 8-1   Distribution of percentage of traumata in relation to age among 9,665 children with traumatic injuries. (From Ravn JJ.[2])

and 9 years (Fig. 8-1).[2-4] Most of the injuries involve the maxillary incisors.[2-4] Boys are injured twice as often as girls.[2,4] Patients with an increased overjet have a significantly greater risk of dental injuries. A study has shown that an increase of the overjet from 0 to 3 mm to 3 to 6 mm doubles the amount of traumatic dental injuries. With an overjet exceeding 6 mm the risk is tripled.[5] An additional trauma factor is insufficient lip closure, which often leaves the maxillary incisors unprotected.[2] Patients treated for dental injuries often sustain repeated trauma to the teeth.[2] Dental injuries

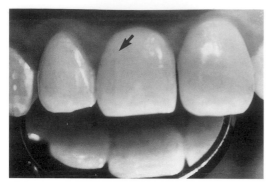

Fig. 8-2   Infraction lines *(arrow)* can be detected by varying the direction of light through the crown with a mirror.

of the primary teeth most often occur at 2 to 4 years of age.[4] There is a close connection between the apices of the primary and secondary teeth. This means that trauma to a primary tooth may cause deformities and eruption disturbances of a secondary tooth.

Fractured teeth

Crown and crown-root fractures

A crown infraction means a fracture of enamel of the tooth only. Such fractures may sometimes be difficult to recognize in direct light, but it is easier if the direction of the light is varied and if at the same time a part of the enamel surface is shaded with a finger (Fig. 8-2).[6] The easiest way to detect infractions is to use fiber optics for the illumination. The presence of infraction lines needs no particular clinical treatment but draws the attention to an earlier trauma. In a study by Ravn,[7] pulp deaths in teeth with infractions caused by concussion accounted for 3.5% of 1,337 incisors.

An uncomplicated crown fracture means a fracture of the crown of the tooth without pulpal involvement. Such a fracture has no immediate effect on the pulp. If the fracture goes both through enamel and dentin and the dentin is left unprotected, a large number of dentinal tubules are opened for invasion of bacteria and toxins. They may cause inflammation of the pulp. The reaction of the pulp depends on the distance between the exposed dentin surface and the pulp and the time of exposure. If the dentin exposure is more severe, the risk is still small for pulpal complications if the dentin surface is properly protected. A study by Stålhane and Hedegård[8] showed that out of 1,546 teeth with crown fractures, only 5 (0.3%) developed pulpal necrosis (Tables 8-1 and 8-2). The prognosis for uncomplicated crown fractures and crown-root fractures is therefore good.[8]

Clinically it is essential that even teeth with small injuries such as infractions and uncomplicated crown fractures are tested for vitality and that a radiographic examination is performed before orthodontic treatment is initiated. When in doubt of the clinical condition of the pulp, a 3-month observation period after the trauma with repeated vitality tests is recommended before orthodontic treatment.

A complicated crown fracture means a fracture involving enamel, dentin, and exposed pulp. If the fracture also involves the root, it is called a *complicated crown-root fracture*.

Healing of a complicated crown fracture or crown-root fracture does not occur spontaneously. Untreated pulpal exposures usually lead to pulpal necrosis. Capping of the pulp with calcium hydroxide or

Table 8-1 Incidence of pulpal complications after traumatic injuries to permanent teeth, as expressed in number of teeth (from Stålhane I and Hedegård[8] B)

Initial diagnosis	No (%) complications	Obliteration (%)	Necrosis (%)	Total no. teeth
Crown fracture	1535 (99.3)	6 (0.4)	5 (0.3)	1546
Subluxation	851 (83.7)	48 (4.7)	119 (11.6)	1018
Luxation	26 (26.4)	19 (19.5)	53 (54.1)	98

Table 8-2 Incidence of root resorption after traumatic injuries to permanent teeth as expressed in number of teeth (from Stålhane I and Hedegård[8] B)

Initial conditions of teeth	No (%) resorptions	Superficial resorption (%)	Progressive resorption (%)	Total no. teeth
Crown fracture	1539 (99.6)	6 (0.4)	1 (0.0)	1546
Subluxation	995 (97.7)	15 (1.5)	8 (0.8)	1018
Luxation	81 (82.8)	9 (9.1)	8 (8.1)	98

partial pulpotomy followed by a calcium hydroxide cover of the pulp can preserve vitality.[9]

In immature teeth it is recommended that the orthodontic movement of the injured teeth be postponed until tooth development is completed or at least until a continued root development is seen. Clinical and radiographic checks are carried out after 6 months, 1 year, and 2 years. In teeth with pulp necrosis it is advisable to wait until the root canal has been filled with gutta-percha after initial treatment with calcium hydroxide.

Root fractures

Orthodontic management of root-fractured teeth depends on the type of healing and location of the fracture (Fig. 8-3). Radiographic and histologic observations have shown different types of healing after a root-fracture, ie, healing with calcified tissue and with connective tissue sometimes combined with ingrowth of bone.[10–12]

Healing with calcified tissue means that the fracture is healed with cementum. The bridging of the fracture may not be completed, but the fracture is consolidated and there is no sign of perapical rounding of the fracture edges. The pulp is partially or totally obliterated. The tooth mobility is nor-

135

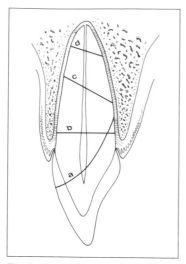

Fig. 8-3   Different locations of root fractures and crown-root fractures. *(a)* Crown-root fracture; *(b)* cervical root fracture; *(c)* middle third root fracture; *(d)* apical third root fracture.

mal and the response to a vitality test is normal or slightly decreased.[10-12]

Orthodontic movement of a root-fractured tooth healed with a hard tissue callus can usually be performed without breaking up the fracture site (Figs. 8-4a to g).

Healing with interposition of connective tissue means that the fracture edges are covered with cementum. A common finding is peripheral roundings of the fracture edges. Often an ingrowth of bone between the fragment can be observed.[13]

Movement of a fractured tooth where the fragments are separated by connective tissue leads to further separation of the fragment. A common finding after treatment is rounding of the coronal fragment (Figs. 8-5a to c). In planning orthodontic therapy it must therefore be realized that a

fractured root with interposition of connective tissue should be looked upon as a tooth with a short root. As a result, such a tooth must be evaluated with respect to the length of the coronal fragment. This means that teeth with fractures in the apical third of the root (Fig. 8-3, *d*) generally have enough root length to allow orthodontic movement. Teeth with fractures located in the middle third of the root (Fig. 8-3, *c*) represent a hazard for orthodontic movement because of the risk for further shortening of the very short coronal fragment. The orthodontic movement may result in a root with very little periodontal support. In cervical root fractures (Figs. 8-3, *a, b*) the apical fragment can sometimes be extruded with a rapid orthodontic extrusion technique or an intraalveolar transplantation (which will be discussed elsewhere in this chapter).

Several clinical studies have demonstrated successful healing of root-fractured teeth, but it has also been reported that 20 % to 22 % develop pulpal necrosis.[11] The coronal fragment of such teeth is often dislocated, and inflammatory changes occur along the fracture lines. Radiographically a widening of the fracture line is seen and clinically the teeth are somewhat mobile, often slightly extruded, and sensitive to percussion. In most cases the pulp in the apical fragment remains vital. Endodontic treatment of the coronal fragment, eg, root filling with gutta percha after initial treatment with calcium hydroxide, seems to offer a good prognosis.[14] If the pulp in the coronal fragment is necrotic and left untreated, the apical fragment may later also become necrotic. Such a fragment must be surgically extracted.

Movement of fractured teeth with a proper root filling may be performed with an equal prognosis as if the coronal fragment is vital.

Figs. 8-4a to g   Orthodontic movement of a root-fractured incisor healed with hard tissue callus. The patient was treated with an activator and extraoral traction for 2 years. Note that the tooth movement was performed without breaking up the fracture site. (From Andreasen, chapter 11.[1])

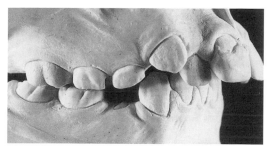
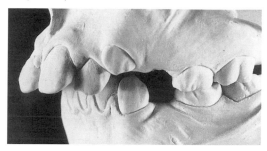

Figs. 8-4a and b   Models of the malocclusion — a Class II, division 1 deep bite, pretreatment.

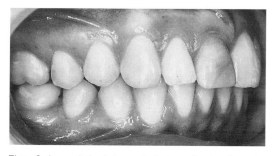
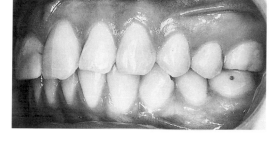

Figs. 8-4c and d   Intraoral photos after treatment.

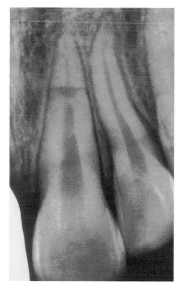
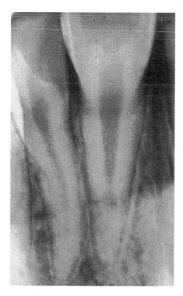
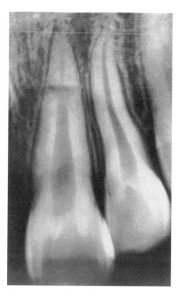

Fig. 8-4e   The root-fractured tooth before treatment.

Fig. 8-4f   Tooth immediately after active treatment.

Fig. 8-4g   Condition of tooth 4 years after treatment.

Figs. 8-5a to c   Orthodontic movement of an incisor with a root fracture healed with interposition of connective tissue. The orthodontic treatment was similar to that in Figs. 8-4a to g.

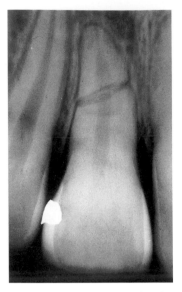 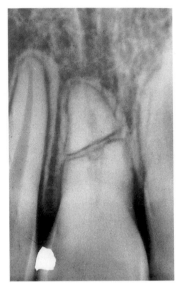 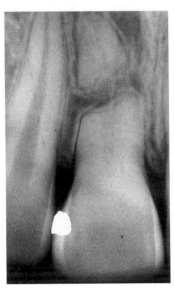

Fig. 8-5a   Two months after the trauma. Note the rounding of the fracture edges.

Fig. 8-5b   After an observation period of 2 years. A further rounding of the fracture edges can be seen.

Fig. 8-5c After orthodontic movement. The fragments have separated with ingrowth of bone.

Observation period

An observation period of 2 years has been recommended before movement of root fractured teeth.[13] Later clinical experience, however, indicates that most of the complications, eg, pulpal necrosis, occur during the first year after the trauma.[15] This means that the observation period may be shortened if no complication occurs. If endodontic treatment is to be performed, orthodontic movement should be postponed until completion of the endodontic therapy and clinical and radiographic evidence of healing are seen.

Orthodontic treatment of fractured teeth

Root fractures

Figures 8-6a to k illustrate the orthodontic movement of two fractured central incisors in a 12-year-old girl. The left central incisor was healed by hard tissue callus (Figs. 8-6i and k) and the right with interposition of connective tissue (Figs. 8-6h and j).

After fixation and an observation period of 2 years a minimal rounding of the fracture edges was evident in the left incisor (Fig. 8-6k). In the right incisor (Fig. 8-6j), the rounding of the fracture edges was more marked. A tendency toward obliteration of

Figs. 8-6a to k   Orthodontic movement of two fractured incisors in a 12-year-old girl with a Class II, division 1 malocclusion. The orthodontic treatment was performed with a modified activator during the late mixed dentition to take advantage of the mandibular growth during this period. An inactive torquing spring was used to avoid lingual tipping of the fractured incisors. The first premolar was extracted and treatment was completed with an edgewise appliance in the permanent dentition. Total treatment time was 2 years.

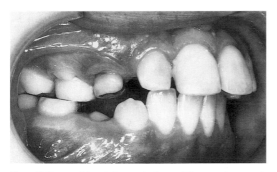
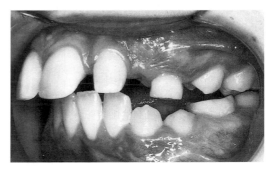

Figs. 8-6a and b   Intraoral view of the postnormal occlusion before treatment.

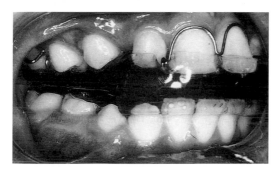

Figs. 8-6c   The modified activator.

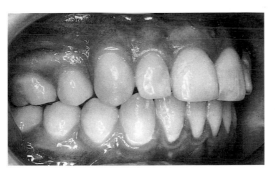
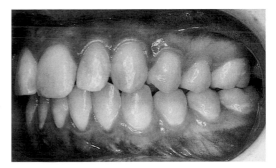

Figs. 8-6d and e   The occlusion after treatment with fixed appliance.

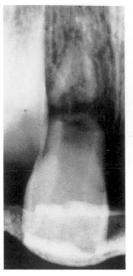
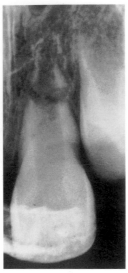
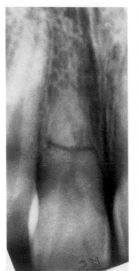
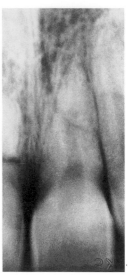

Figs. 8-6f and g Radiographs immediately after the trauma. The teeth were splinted with an acrylic splint for about 8 weeks.

Figs. 8-6h and i Two years after the trauma. Root development has continued in both of the central incisors. The fracture of the right central incisor is healed with interposition of connective tissue between the fracture edges. In the left central incisor a hard tissue callus can be seen.

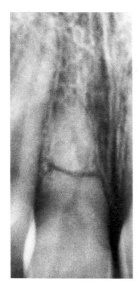
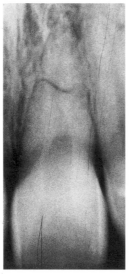

Figs. 8-6j and k Radiographs 2 years after active treatment. There is a marked rounding of the fracture edges in the right central incisor with a wide fracture line. In the left central incisor the fracture edges are not affected by the tooth movement. There is a normal tooth mobility of the left incisor but the mobility of the right incisor is a little increased.

the coronal pulps can be seen. During the orthodontic movement a further rounding of the fracture edges was seen in the right incisor (Fig. 8-6j), while the fracture in the left incisor was not affected by the tooth movement (Fig. 8-6k). Both teeth are still vital, and there is no widening of the periodontal contours around the apical fragments. There is some mobility in the left incisor.

Crown-root fractures and cervical root fractures

To complete a crown restoration on a tooth with a complicated crown-root fracture where the fracture line goes below the marginal bone level, it is often necessary to extrude the root. Two types of therapy are available, orthodontic extrusion[16-21, 60] and surgical intraalveolar transplantation.[22-24] The exact indications for the two alternatives have not yet been elucidated.

Orthodontic extrusion

In the case of complicated fracture with pulpal involvement, endodontic therapy should be performed before orthodontic treatment.[16, 17] This endodontic treatment is often difficult to perform under sterile conditions without gingivectomy. At the surgical exposure of the fracture edges it is important to explore further fractures. Special attention should be paid to the lingual part of the root (Fig. 8-7). A step in this part might indicate further fractures. Axial fractures should also be carefully explored after the gingivectomy.

When endodontic treatment is completed and apical healing is seen, a cast core is made with a separate temporary crown. In the cervical part of the cast core a hole is made (Fig. 8-8a). This hole also

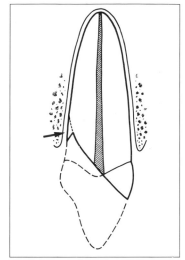

Fig. 8-7   Before orthodontic extrusion is performed, special attention should be paid to the lingual part of the root to explore fractures reaching deep below the marginal bone level *(arrow)*.

goes through the temporary crown (Fig. 8-8b). A steel ligature wire is threaded through the hole. The ligature is used to fasten a spring to the tooth. When it is not possible to make a cast core, a steel hook

Fig. 8-8a   A cast core with a hole for orthodontic extrusion. (From Malmgren et al.[60])

Fig. 8-8b   The hole also goes through the temporary crown. Note that the cast must be short to allow extrusion of the root.

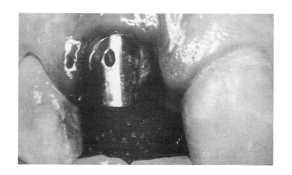

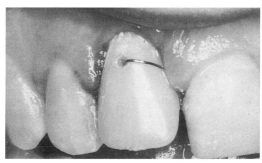

Figs. 8-9a to f   Rapid orthodontic extrusion of the left central incisor with a crown-root fracture. The fracture line goes below the alveolar bone level. Treatment was performed to facilitate a bridge therapy from teeth 12 to 21 and lasted for 3 weeks. The retention period was 1 month.

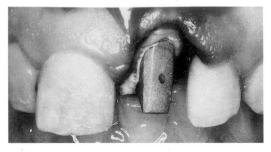
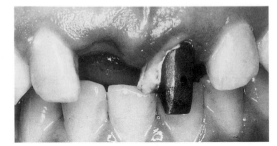

Figs. 8-9a and b   The root with a cast core before and after the extrusion. Note the change of the gingival contour.

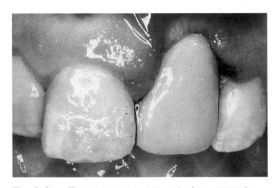
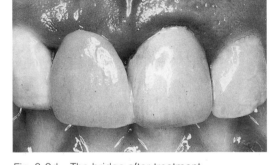

Fig. 8-9c   The temporary crown before extrusion.   Fig. 8-9d   The bridge after treatment.

Figs. 8-9e and f   Radiographs before and after the rapid extrusion.

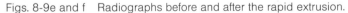

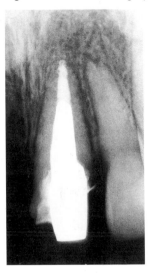
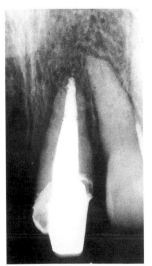

can be cemented in the root canal. Sometimes it is even possible to bond a button on enamel remnants of the crown. The orthodontic extrusion is normally carried out over a period of 3 to 4 weeks.[18] The extrusion leads to a coronal shift of the marginal gingiva. It has been shown that this gingival shift consists of an increase of the attached gingiva and not only by coronal displacement.[18] The orthodontic extrusion should therefore in most cases be followed by a gingivectomy (Figs. 8-9a–f).

It is well known that rapid extrusion of vital teeth can cause pulpal damage.[24] Teeth with a severe crown-root fracture are nearly always nonvital and root filled and can be extruded rapidly, 3 to 5 mm in 3 or 4 weeks.[16, 18] The rapid extrusion is possible because the tooth movement is accomplished by stretching and readjustment of periodontal fibers and not by bone remodeling. The rapid extrusion can thus be done without coronal shift of marginal bone, which facilitates the crown restoration, because no subsequent bone remodeling is necessary. Rapid orthodontic extrusion compared to normal orthodontic movement raises the question of damage to the root. Histologic studies of extruded human teeth[23] and clinical experience indicate that root resorption is very rare.

Relapse can occur after orthodontic extrusion. A retention period of 6 months has been recommended.[19] The prime reason for the relapse is stretching of the marginal periodontal fibers. Clinical experience indicates that fibrotomy immediately after the extrusion lessens the risk for relapse and that a retention period of only 3 to 4 weeks is necessary (Figs. 8-10a–g, page 144).

A tooth with an uncomplicated crown-root fracture and vital pulp should be extruded slowly, 2 or 3 mm in 4 to 8 months, in order to protect the vitality of the pulp. It is then often necessary to recontour both the marginal gingiva and the bone.[24]

Surgical intraalveolar transplantation

Intraalveolar transplantation is a method for surgical extrusion of crown-root fractured teeth. The method is recommended when further fractures of the root are suspected. The root can easily be inspected during the transplantation. Root filling can be performed after the extrusion. Sometimes it is also advisable to rotate the root, thereby reducing extrusion and facilitating crown therapy. A surgical technique for the intraalveolar transplantation is described by Tegsjö et al[25] (Figs. 8-11a–i, page 145).

A mucoperiostal flap is raised buccally from the tooth. Bone is then removed from the apical area at the height of the root apex. The root is luxated with a crown remover with falling weight and extruded until the entire fracture line is clinically accessible. The bone that is removed from the apical area is modeled with a nipper and wedged in as a support apically to the root. The flap is sutured with single sutures over the alveolus as a support to the root.

A simpler surgical technique is to perform the extrusion after carefully mobilizing the root with elevators and cutting the marginal periodontal fibers with a sharp carver. Immobilization of the root after extrusion is achieved with interdental sutures on both sides of the extruded root (Figs. 8-12a to e, page 146).[26-28]

In comparison to surgical extrusion, the orthodontic method seems to give a minimal risk for root resorption and a favorable

Figs. 8-10a to g   Rapid extrusion of a crown-root fractured right central incisor. The fractured crown was temporarily fixed to the root with a screw-post. (From Malmgren et al.[60])

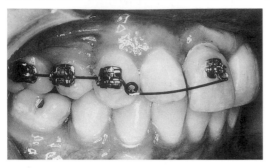

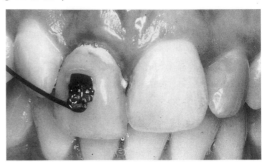

Fig. 8-10a   A stainless steel spring (.016 x .016) with an extrusion force of about 60 p was used.

Fig. 8-10b   After 1 week the tooth was extruded 1.5 mm.

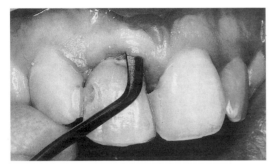

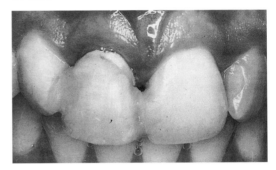

Figs. 8-10c and d   After 3 weeks the tooth was extruded about 3 mm. (Left) A gingivectomy and a fibrotomy were performed. The extruded tooth was splinted to the neighboring teeth for 1 month. Thereafter a permanent crown was made. (Right)

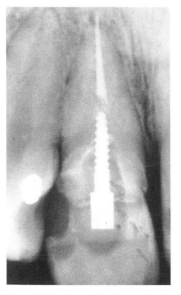

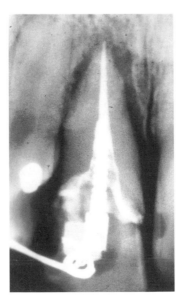

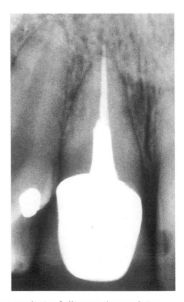

Figs. 8-10e to g   Radiographs before and immediately after the extrusion and at a followup 1 year later.

Figs. 8-11a to i   Surgical intraalveolar transplantation. (From Tegsjö et al.[25])

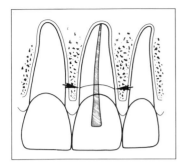

Fig. 8-11a   A cervical root fracture with the fracture line below the marginal bone level *(arrows).*

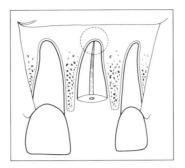

Fig. 8-11b   A mucoperiosteal flap is raised buccally of the tooth. Bone is then removed from the apical area at the height of the root apex *(circle).*

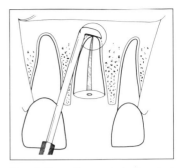

Fig. 8-11c   The root is luxated with a crown remover with a falling weight.

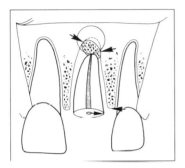

Fig. 8-lld   The bone that has been removed from the apical area is wedged in as a support to the root *(arrows).*

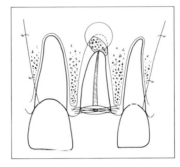

Fig. 8 11e   The flap is sutured with single sutures, two of which are placed in a cross over the alveolus.

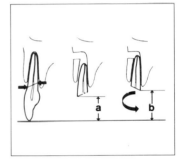

Fig. 8-11f   The root can be rotated to minimize the degree of extrusion.

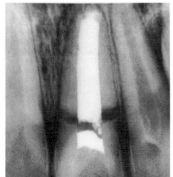

Fig. 8-11g   A cervical root fracture in the left central incisor situated 2 mm below the bone margin. The tooth has been previously root filled in connection with an earlier trauma.

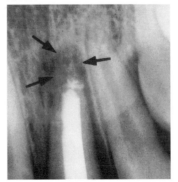

Fig. 8-11h   Immediately postoperatively. The bone transplant is indicated by arrows.

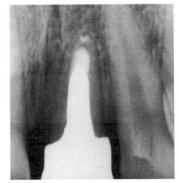

Fig. 8-11i   After 1 year. The periapical bone structure and the periodontal space is normal.

Figs. 8-12a to e   A simplified surgical intraalveolar transplantation technique. (From Kahnberg.[27])

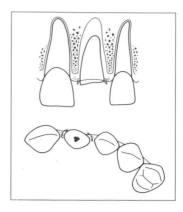

Fig. 8-12a   The extrusion is performed by carefully mobilizing the root with elevators and cutting off the marginal periodontal fibers with a sharp carver. Immobilization is achieved with interdental sutures on both sides of the extruded root.

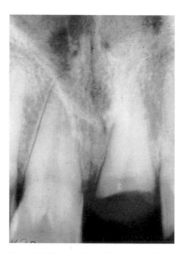

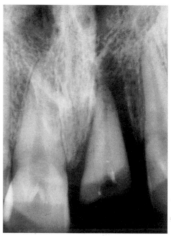

Figs. 8-12b and c   Preoperative radiographs of the left central incisor with a cervical root fracture.

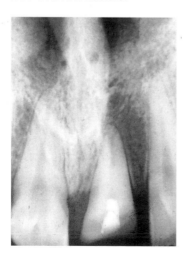

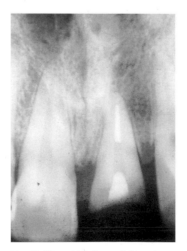

Fig. 8-12d   One week after surgical extrusion.

Fig. 8-12e   Healing of the alveolus 3 months postoperatively.

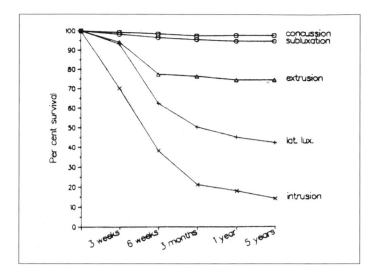

Fig. 8-13   Pulp survival after luxation injuries. Estimates of survival without pulp necrosis of teeth in five luxation categories based on 400 patients with 637 luxated permanent teeth. (From Andreasen and Vestergard-Pedersen.[35])

gingival contour. The excess of gingiva after the orthodontic extrusion can be re-contoured to fit the crown. The surgical technique is recommended (1) when the fracture edges are more than 3 to 4 mm below the marginal bone level; (2) when endodontic therapy is impossible before extrusion; (3) when further fractures of the root are suspected; and (4) when a rotation of the root is preferable. The surgical procedure has so far proved to involve relatively few complications. A success rate of 71% to 85% has been reported[28, 29] without progressive root resorptions or other pathologic complications.

Luxated teeth

When a tooth is dislocated in the alveolus by a traumatic force both the periodontal structures and the blood supply of the pulp are influenced. The damage to the structures depends on the degree and direction of the force. A concussion means an injury without abnormal loosening or displacement of the tooth, but the tooth has a marked reaction to percussion. Subluxation means an injury with abnormal loosening of the tooth without displacement. Intrusion, extrusion, and lateral luxation mean displacement of the tooth in respective directions. Exarticulation means a complete avulsion of the tooth out of its socket.[30-35]

Minor injuries such as concussions, subluxations, and small extrusions often have an uncomplicated healing and the damage of the cementum and dentin is repaired with cementum. The healing events of severe injuries, such as intrusions, lateral luxations, and exarticulations followed by replantation of the teeth, are more complicated. The risk for pulpal necrosis[31, 32, 35] and root resorption is greater (Fig. 8-13).[1] Such complications are particularly evident in replanted teeth. The extraalveolar period and the type of storage media used are the

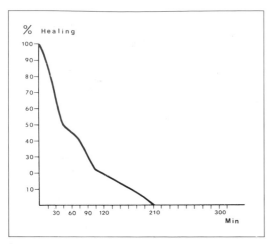

% Healing

Min

Fig. 8-14 Relationship between the extraoral period before replantation and the radiographic occurrence of inflammatory and replacement resorption in 110 replanted human teeth. (From Andreasen and Hjörting-Hansen.[37])

most important factors for the prognosis (Fig. 8-14).[36–39]

Root resorption

Damage to the periodontal structure can result in three types of external root resorptions: surface resorption, inflammatory resorption or replacement resorption.

Surface resorption means a superficial resorption that is repaired with new cementum. Teeth with minor resorptions can be moved orthodontically with a prognosis similar to that of uninjured teeth.[40]

Inflammatory resorption means a rapid resorption of both cementum and dentin with inflammation of adjacent periodontal tissue. This type of resorption is related to an infected and necrotic pulp. The resorptions are usually seen 3 to 6 weeks after an injury.[32, 33] It is essential that proper

endodontic treatment is initiated as soon as possible. The necrotic pulp tissue is extirpated and a temporary root filling with calcium hydroxide is placed. Arrest of the inflammatory resorption can be seen in about 96% of cases after this treatment.[14] Orthodontic treatment should be postponed until radiographic signs of healing are seen.

Teeth with signs of root resorption after endodontic treatment seem to be more susceptible to further resorption during orthodontic movement.[40] This does not necessarily contraindicate the treatment, but special care should be taken to avoid excessive pressure during movement.

Replacement resorption or *ankylosis* means a direct union between bone and root substance. This type of resorption is progressive: the periodontal space disappears and successively the whole root disappears.[1, 36] The rate of this resorption varies individually, and in many cases the tooth can be used as a space maintainer for several years.

Teeth with replacement resorption do not respond to orthodontic movement. The resorption is most often clinically recognized during the first 2 months after a severe trauma.[37] The tooth becomes immobile, and percussion produces a high sound compared to that of neighboring, uninjured teeth. In radiographs the periodontal space disappears and the root substance is replaced by bone.

In children and adolescents with growing jaws the ankylosed tooth may become infraoccluded and the neighboring teeth often tilt toward it.[37–39] If the patient is in a period of rapid growth and the degree of infraocclusion becomes more than one third of the crown length, there is an indication for extraction of the ankylosed tooth.

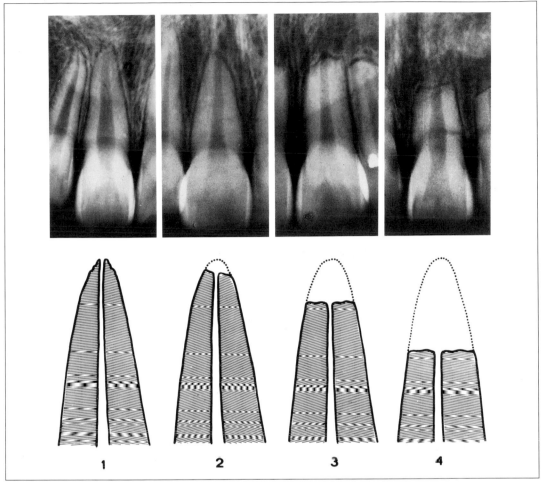

Fig. 8-15   Root resorption index for quantitative assessment of root resorption. *(1)* Irregular root contour; *(2)* root resorption less than 2 mm (minor resorption); *(3)* root resorption apically, from 2 mm to one third of the original root length (severe resorption); *(4)* root resorption exceeding one third of the original root length (extreme resorption). (From Levander and Malmgren.[42])

Special care is then needed to avoid excessive loss of alveolar bone.[41]

Observation periods

There may be different complications after luxation of teeth. Clinical experience indicates an observation period of at least 3 months after a mild injury, eg, concussion, subluxation. After a moderate or severe trauma (extrusion, intrusion, replantation) the observation period should be at least 1 year.

Teeth with repaired superficial resorption or repaired inflammatory resorptions during this observation period should be carefully followed during orthodontic movement. A radiographic study of the roots prior to treatment gives information of some risk factors.[42] It is important to observe teeth with an irregular root contour, concavities along the surface of the root, or root malformations. The risk for root resorption of such teeth during movement is high. It is necessary to make regular radiographic checks in order to detect whether any root resorption is occurring. An index provides a useful tool for quantitative assessment of root conditions during treatment (Fig. 8-15).

Orthodontic treatment of luxated teeth

Root resorption

Luxated teeth may have a higher risk for root resorption during orthodontic treatment than uninjured teeth, particularly if there has been damage to the root cementum.[40] However, the etiology of root resorption is a complicated question, and there is no single explanation as to why certain teeth resorb severely during orthodontic treatment. Instead, a number of cumulative factors may explain why resorption takes place. Most authors consider heavy forces responsible for root resorption.[43-46] Intensity and duration of forces are of great importance. Heavy forces of continuous duration can also cause resorption.[47] Prolonged tipping of a tooth can cause root resorption as well as resorption of the alveolar crest, especially in adult patients.[56]

A study has shown that the risk for severe root resorption can, to a certain degree, be estimated after 6 to 9 months of treatment with a fixed appliance.[42] Signs of

root resorption were registered with index scores from 0 to 4. The risk for severe resorption (a score of 3 or 4) was described as minimal, small, moderate, or high if the percentage of roots in a studied group with such resorptions was 0%, 0% to 25%, 25% to 50%, and 50%, respectively.

A severe resorption noted after 6 to 9 months of treatment was found to indicate a high risk for extreme resorption, a small resorption a moderate risk, and an irregular root contour a small risk for severe resorption (Fig. 8-16). If no resorption was noted, the risk for severe resorption at the end of treatment was minimal. It was also found that there was a high risk for severe root resorption if the roots were pipette shaped and a moderate risk if they were blunt (Fig. 8-17).

It is important to start treatment of luxated teeth with light forces.[48] It is also advisable to make a check after 3 to 4 months. A small resorption at this check indicates a risk for further resorption at the end of treatment and a severe resorption a high risk for an extreme resorption. If the check shows a risk for severe root resorption, the aims of treatment should be reevaluated.

During treatment, movement of teeth into cortical bone should be avoided.[49] If the alveolar crest is narrow, it is easy to move proclined or retroclined maxillary incisors into labial or lingual cortical bone. To avoid this it is advisable to perform the root movement by first intruding the roots into the cancellous bone area and then moving the teeth (Figs. 8-18a to c).

Intrusion of permanent teeth

Intrusion of a permanent tooth into the alveolar bone is a severe traumatic injury.

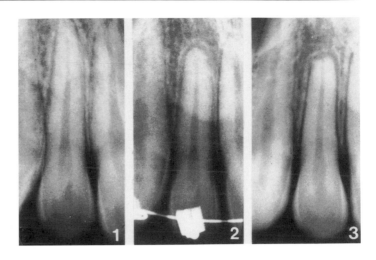

Fig. 8-16 Root resorption after treatment with fixed appliance in relation to initial resorption after 6 to 9 months. *(1)* Before treatment; *(2)* after 6 months minor resorption can be seen; *(3)* at the end of complete orthodontic treatment with fixed appliance. (From Levander and Malmgren.[42])

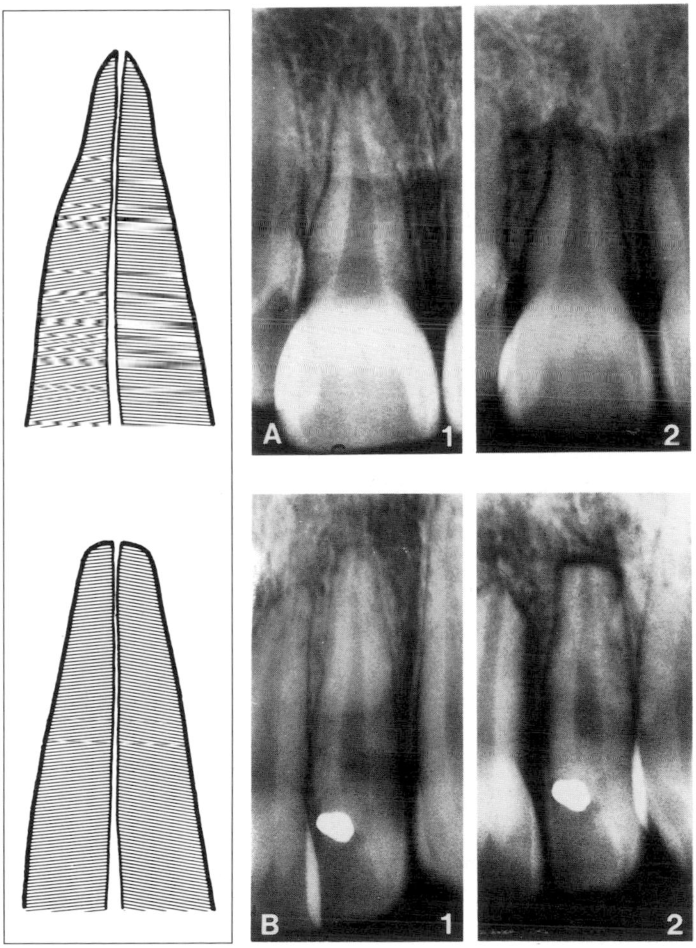

Fig. 8-17 Typical effect of root resorption on teeth with deviating root forms.
(A) A pipette-shaped root *(1)* before and *(2)* after treatment with fixed appliance.
(B) A blunt root *(1)* before and *(2)* after treatment with fixed appliance. (From Levander and Malmgren.[42])

151

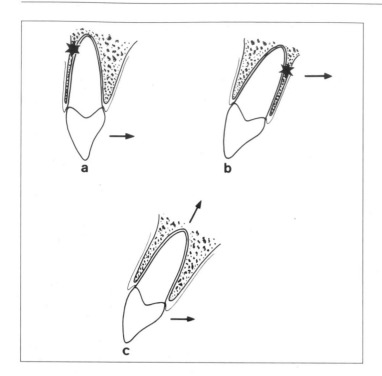

Figs. 8-18 *(a and b)* Lingual tipping of incisors moves the root into contact with the buccal cortical plate, and lingual torque can move it into the palatal cortical plate. The contact can cause root resorption. *(c)* Intrusion of incisors into the roomier cancellous part of the bone area before lingual tipping or torquing is used to avoid the contact with the cortical plate (From Ten Hoeve and Mulie.[49])

Periodontal damage can cause ankylosis, root resorption, pulpal necrosis, pulpal obliteration, and loss of marginal bone support.[35, 50] The risks for ankylosis and pulpal damage are important factors in the plan of treatment.

The risk for these complications is less in intruded immature teeth, which may be left to erupt spontaneously if the intrusion is not too severe (Figs. 8-19a to g).[51]

In mature teeth there is a great risk for pulpal damage.[35] Endodontic treatment is necessary in most cases. A necrotic and infected pulp can lead to rapid inflammatory root resorption.[52] The critical period for the start of such external resorption after the intrusion is 2 to 3 weeks.

To facilitate the endodontic therapy and minimize the risk for root resorption and ankylosis, the intruded tooth has to be re-positioned within the first weeks after the injury. This can be done by orthodontic or surgical therapy.[1, 53–57] Andreasen[1] recommends orthodontic extrusion, reporting more complications such as root resorption and loss of marginal support after surgical repositioning (Figs. 8-20a to h). An experimental study in dogs, however, has shown that orthodontic extrusion has little effect if the intrusion is severe.[57] Another factor is that after a severe intrusion there is a risk that the tooth is tightly secured within the bone. The orthodontic forces may not overcome this mechanical barrier. There may also be direct contact between the cementum and bone because of the damage to the periodontium. This can accelerate the development of ankylosis and make orthodontic extrusion impossible.[57] To avoid these complications a luxation of the

Figs. 8-19a to g   An intruded immature left central incisor in a 6-year-old boy. The tooth was left to erupt spontaneously.

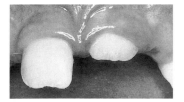

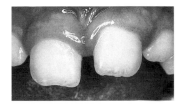

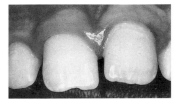

Fig. 8-19a   Immediately after the extrusion.

Fig. 8-19b   After 6 months.

Fig. 8-19c   After 2 years.

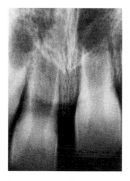

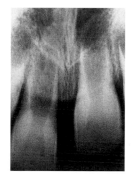

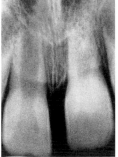

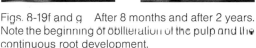

Fig. 8-19d   Radiograph immediately after the trauma.

Fig. 8-19e   After 4 months.

Figs. 8-19f and g   After 8 months and after 2 years. Note the beginning of obliteration of the pulp and the continuous root development.

intruded tooth can be performed before the orthodontic extrusion (Figs. 8-20a to h). Severe intrusions are often accompanied by fractures of the alveolar walls. If an immediate surgical extrusion is performed, the fracture edges of the alveolar walls can be repositioned at the same time (Figs. 8-21a to o, pages 155 to 158).

As a clinical guideline, teeth with severe intrusive injuries should be surgically repositioned, whereas those with less severe intrusion should be orthodontically extruded. If the teeth are tightly secured within the bone, a slight luxation and extrusion facilitates the orthodontic therapy.

Replanted and transplanted teeth

In patients where an exarticulated tooth has been replanted it may be advisable to move the replanted tooth orthodontically. No report concerning the effect of orthodontic treatment upon replanted teeth seems to be available. Most of the complications after the replantation, such as inflammatory resorption and ankylosis, occur during the first year after the trauma.[36, 37] According to the author's experience, if no such complication is seen, movement of a replanted tooth is possible without severe resorptions.

Good prognoses following autotransplantation of premolars to replace missing

Figs. 8-20a to h   Intruded maxillary central incisors in a 6-year-old boy. The teeth were tightly stuck in the bone. First they were loosened and slightly extruded by digital pressure, keeping the fingers over the apical area. They were then extruded by orthodontic springs. (From Andreasen, chapter 11.[1])

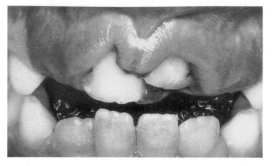

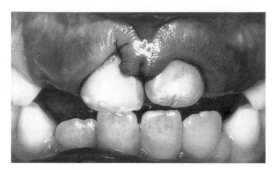

Figs. 8-20a to h   Intruded maxillary central incisors in a 6-year-old boy. The teeth were tightly stuck in the bone. First they were loosened and slightly extruded by digital pressure, keeping the fingers over the apical area. They were then extruded by orthodontic springs.

Fig. 8-20b   After loosening and a slight extrusion with fingers.

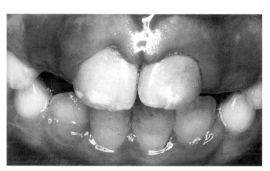

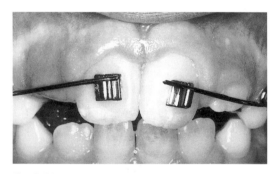

Fig. 8-20c   After 2 weeks.

Fig. 8-20d   A plate with extrusion springs.

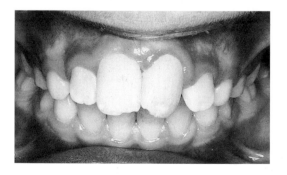

Fig. 8-20e   After orthodontic extrusion.

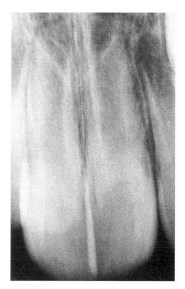

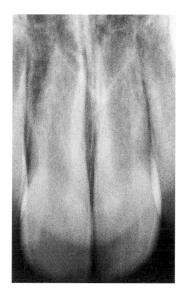

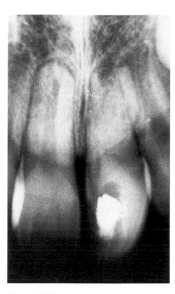

Fig. 8-20f Radiograph immediately after the trauma.

Fig. 8-20g After orthodontic extrusion.

Fig. 8-20h Endodontic therapy
initiated in tooth 21; 11 is vital.

Figs. 8-21a to o A severe trauma in a 10-year-old girl: tooth 11 is intruded and tooth 21 is exarticulated. Tooth 21 was replanted some minutes after the trauma, and tooth 11 was surgically repositioned. There was a fracture of the alveolar wall. The fracture sites were repositioned. The anterior teeth were splinted with a twistflex arch for 3 weeks. Endodontic therapy was initiated 2 weeks after the trauma. A temporary root filling of teeth 11 and 21 using calcium hydroxide was performed. A permanent root filling with gutta percha was done 1 year after the trauma. The girl had a Class II, division 1 malocclusion. Two months after the trauma, an extraoral traction with headgear and bands on teeth 16 and 26 was started. After 1 year, treatment with a fixed appliance and Class II traction was initiated. Total treatment time was 2 years. (From Malmgren et al.[41])

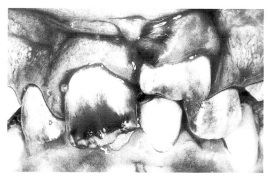

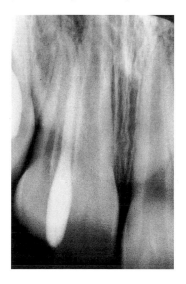

Fig. 8-21a Immediately after the trauma, tooth 11 was intruded and tooth 21 exarticulated and re-planted.

Fig. 8-21b Radiograph of tooth 11 immediately after the trauma.

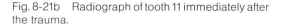

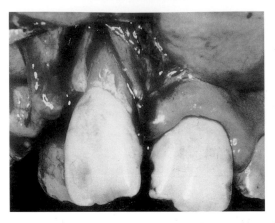
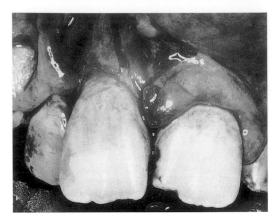

Figs. 8-21c and d   Tooth 11 was surgically repositioned and a fracture of the alveolar wall buccal of tooth 11 was repositioned at the same time.

Figs. 8-21e to g   Splinting of the incisors with a twistflex arch.

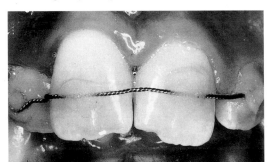

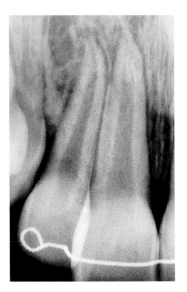
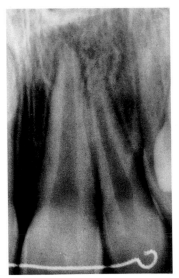

Figs. 8-21h to j   Two months after the trauma treatment with headgear was started. After 1 year treatment with a fixed appliance was initiated.

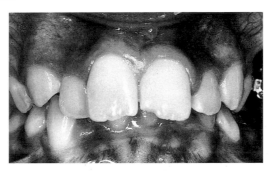

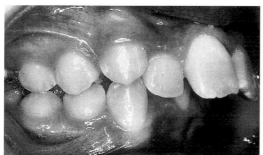
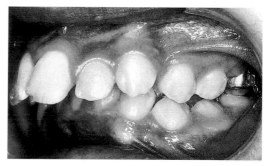

Figs. 8-21k to m   After treatment with the fixed appliance.

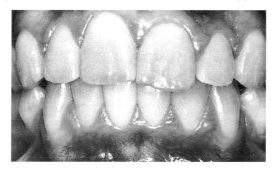

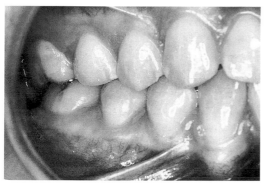
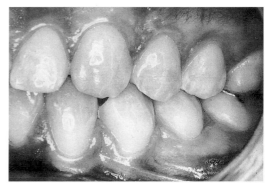

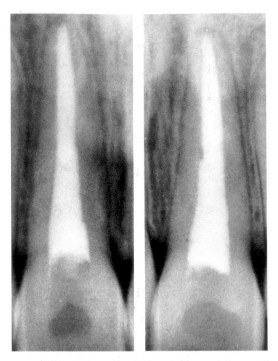

Figs. 8-21n and o   Teeth 11 and 21 at a followup 2 years after orthodontic treatment and 4 years after the trauma.

in the actual position as a space maintainer until complete resorption has occurred. If it has to be extracted prior to the orthodontic treatment or during the initial stages, there is a great risk for extensive loss of alveolar bone at the extraction site.

To avoid such bone loss a new technique for extraction has been described.[41] The method involves removal of the crown and the root filling from the ankylosed root. The root is then covered with a mucoperiosteal flap (Figs. 8-22a to l). It has been shown that it is possible with this method to preserve the alveolar bone around the ankylosed root. The condition for the subsequent orthodontic or prosthetic therapy is improved (Figs. 8-23a to d).

incisors have been reported. Several reports conclude that autotransplantation has the best results when a tooth germ has developed one half to three fourths of the complete root length.[58] It has also been shown that transplanted teeth can be moved with only a minor shortening of the root length.[59]

Complications

If, after a severe luxation, injury, or replantation a tooth is ankylosed, it cannot be moved orthodontically. When an ankylosis is diagnosed it must therefore be decided whether to extract the tooth or to maintain it

Figs. 8-22a to l   Surgical treatment of ankylosed teeth. (From Malmgren et al.[41])

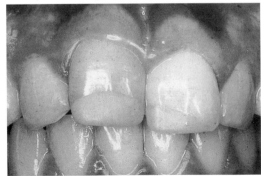

Fig. 8-22a   An ankylosed right central incisor before treatment.

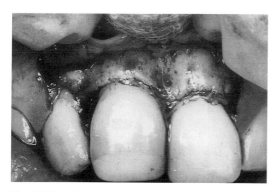

Fig. 8-22b   A marginal incision is made palatally, followed by loosening of the periosteum from the alveolar bone. Buccally, a marginal incision is extended over adjacent teeth and continued at a right angle over the alveolar crest. A buccal mucoperiosteal flap is raised.

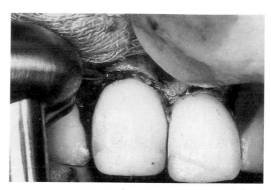

Fig. 8-22c   The crown is removed at the cemento-enamel junction with a diamond bur in an air turbine handpiece, using water spray.

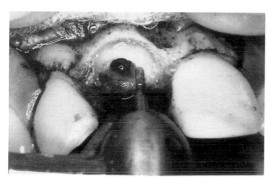

Fig. 8-22d   The root surface is ground down to a level 1.5 to 2 mm below the edge of the marginal bone. This is done with a cylindrical diamond bur during continuous flushing with steril saline.

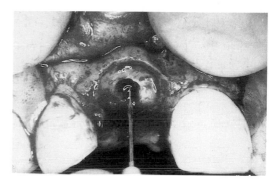

Fig. 8-22e   The root filling is removed with root canal reamers and files. The canal is rinsed with saline.

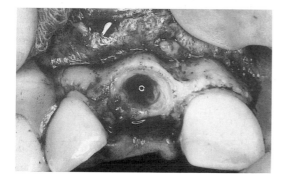

Fig. 8-22f   The canal is allowed to fill with blood.

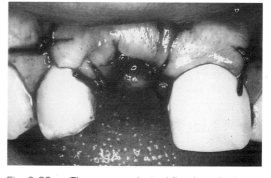

Fig. 8-22g   The mucoperiosteal flap is pulled over the alveolus and sutured with single sutures. It is important that a blood clot is formed in the gap between buccal and palatal mucosa.

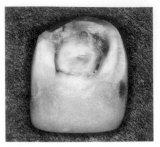
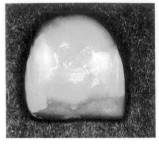
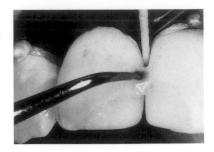

Figs. 8-22h and i   Treatment is completed by remodeling the removed crown with a composite resin.

Fig. 8-22j   The remodeled crown is attached with composite resin to adjacent teeth.

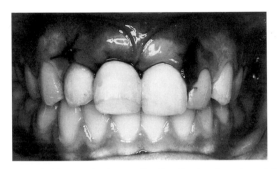
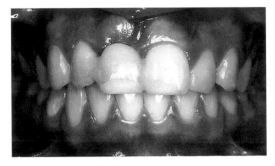

Figs. 8-22k and l   Immediately after treatment and 12 months postoperatively.

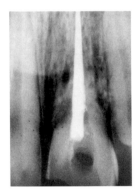
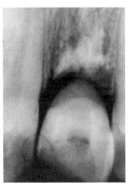
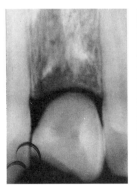
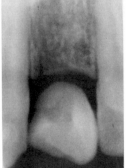

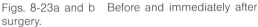

Figs. 8-23a and b   Before and immediately after surgery.

Figs. 8-23c and d   Six and 12 months after surgery. Note the shortened pontic and formation of new bone coronal to root remnants.

References

1. *Andreasen J O. Traumatic Injuries of the Teeth.* 2nd ed. Copenhagen: Munksgaard; 1981.
2. *Ravn J J.* Dental injuries in Copenhagen schoolchildren school year 1967–1972. *Community Dent Oral Epidemiol.* 1974; 2:231–245.
3. *Hedegård B, Stålhane I.* A study of traumatized permanent teeth in children aged 7–15 years. *Swed Dent J* 1973; 66:431–450.
4. *Andreasen J O, Ravn J J.* Epidemiology of traumatic dental injuries to primary and permanent teeth in a Danish population sample. *Int J Oral Surg* 1972; 1:235–239.
5. *Järvinen S.* Incisal overjet and traumatic injuries to upper permanent incisors. A retrospective study. *Acta Odont Scand* 1978; 36:359–362.
6. *Dominkovic T.* Total reflection in tooth substance and diagnosis of cracks in teeth. *Swed Dent J* 1977; 1:163–172.
7. *Ravn J J.* Follow-up study of permanent incisors with enamel cracks as a result of an acute trauma. *Scand J Dent Res* 1981; 89:117–123.
8. *Stålhane I, Hedegård B.* Traumatized permanent teeth in children aged 7–15 years. Part II. *Swed Dent J* 1975; 68:157–169.
9. *Cvek M A.* Clinical report on partial pulpotomy and capping with calcium hydroxide in permanent incisors with complicated crown fracture. *J Endod* 1978; 4:232–237.
10. *Andreasen J O, Hjörting-Hansen E.* Intraalveolar root fractures. Radiographic and histologic study of 50 cases. *J Oral Surg* 1967; 25:414–426.
11. *Zachrisson B U, Jacobson I.* Long term prognosis of 66 permanent anterior teeth with root fracture. *Scand J Dent Res* 1975; 83:345–354.
12. *Jacobsen I, Zachrisson B.* Repair characteristics of root fractures in permanent anterior teeth. *Scand J Dent Res* 1975; 83:355–364.
13. *Zachrisson B U, Jacobsen I.* Response to orthodontic movement of anterior teeth with root fractures. *Trans Eur Orthod Soc* 1974; 44:235–242.
14. *Cvek M. Endodontic treatment of traumatized teeth.* In: Andreasen J O (ed): *Traumatic Injuries of the Teeth.* 2nd ed. Copenhagen: Munskgaard International Publishers; 1981.
15. *Jacobsen I, Kerekes K.* Diagnosis and treatment of pulp necrosis in permanent anterior teeth with root fracture. *Scand J Dent Res* 1980; 88:370–376.
16. *Heithersay G S.* Combined endodontic orthodontic treatment of transverse root fractures in the region of the alveolar crest. *Oral Surg Oral Med Oral Pathol* 1973; 36:404–415.
17. *Wolfson E M, Seiden L.* Combined endodontic-orthodontic treatment of subgingivally fractured teeth. *Can Dent Assoc J* 1975; 11:621–624.
18. *Ingber J S.* Forced eruption: Part II. A method of treating nonrestorable teeth – periodontal and restorative considerations. *J Periodont* 1976; 47:203–216.
19. *Persson M, Serneke D.* Ortodontisk framdragning av tand med cervikal rotfraktur för att möjliggöra kronersättning. *Tandläkartidningen* 1977; 69:1263–1269.
20. *Delivanis P, Delivanis H, Kuftinec M M.* Endodontic-orthodontic management of fractured anterior teeth. *J Am Dent Assoc* 1978; 97:483–485.
21. *Simon J H S, Kelly W H, Gordon D G, Ericksen G W.* Extrusion of endodontically treated teeth. *J Am Dent Assoc* 1978; 97:17–23.
22. *Reitan K.* Clinical and histologic observations on tooth movement during and after orthodontic movement. *Am J Orthod* 1967; 53:721–745.
23. *Reitan K.* Initial tissue behavior during apical root resorption. *Angle Orthod* 1974; 44:68–82.
24. *Oppenheim A.* Artificial elongation of teeth. *Am J Orthod Oral Surg* 1940; 26:931–940.
25. *Tegsjö U, Valerius-Olsson H, Olgart K.* Intraalveolar transplantation of teeth with cervical root fractures. *Swed Dent J* 1978; 2:73–82.
26. *Kahnberg K-E, Warfvinge J, Birgersson B.* Intraalveolar transplantation. The use of antologous bone transplants in the periapical region. *Int J Oral Surg* 1982; 11:372–379.
27. *Kahnberg K-E.* Intraalveolar transplantation of teeth with crown-root fractures. *J Oral Maxillofac Surg* 1985; 43:38–42.
28. *Kahnberg K-E.* Surgical extrusion of root fractured teeth – a follow-up study of two surgical methods. *Endod Dent Traumatol* 1988; 4:85–89.
29. *Tegsjö U, Valerius-Olsson H, Frykholm A, Olgart K.* Clinical evaluation of intraalveolar transplantation of teeth with cervical root fractures. *Swed Dent J* 1987; 11:235–250.
30. *Skieller V.* The prognosis for young injured teeth loosened after mechanical injuries. *Acta Odontol Scand* 1950; 18:171–181.
31. *Eklund G, Stålhane I, Hedegård B.* Traumatized permanent teeth in children aged 7–15 years. Part III. A multivariate analysis of post-traumatic complications of subluxated and luxated teeth. *Swed Dent J* 1976; 69:179–189.
32. *Jacobsen I.* Criteria for diagnosis of pulp necrosis in traumatized permanent incisors. *Scand J Dent Res* 1980; 88:306–312.
33. *Andreasen J O.* Luxation of permanent teeth due to trauma. A clinical and radiographic follow-up study of 189 injured teeth. *Scand J Dent Res* 1970; 78:273–286.

34. *Andreasen F M, Andreasen J O.* Diagnosis of luxation injuries. The importance of standardized clinical radiographic and photographic technique in clinical investigations. *Endod Dent Traumatol* 1985; 1:160–169.

35. *Andreasen F M, Vestergaard-Pedersen B.* Prognosis of luxated permanent teeth – the development of pulp necrosis. *Endod Dent Traumatol* 1985; 1:207–220.

36. *Andreasen J O, Hjörting-Hansen E.* Replantation of teeth. II. Histological study of 22 replanted anterior teeth in humans. *Acta Odontol Scand* 1966; 24:287–306.

37. *Andreasen J O, Hjörting-Hansen E.* Replantation of teeth. I. Radiographic and clinical study of 110 human teeth replanted after accidental loss. *Acta Odontol Scand* 1966; 24:263–286.

38. *Ravn J J, Helbo M.* Replantation af acidentelt eksatikulerede taender. *Tandlaegebladet* 1966; 70:805–815.

39. *Koch G, Ullbro C.* Klinisk funktionstid hos 55 exartikulerade och replanterade tänder. *Tandlaekartidningen.* 1982; 74:18–25.

40. *Malmgren O, Goldson L, Hill C, Orvin A, Petrini L, Lundberg M.* Root resorption after orthodontic treatment of traumatized teeth. *Am J Orthod* 1982; 82:6,487–491.

41. *Malmgren B, Cvek M, Lundberg M, Frykholm A.* Surgical treatment of ankylosed and infrapositioned reimplanted incisors in adolescents. *Scand J Dent Res* 1984; 92:391–399.

42. *Levander E, Malmgren O.* Evaluation of the risk of root resorption during orthodontic treatment: a study of upper incisors. *Eur J Orthod* 1988; 10:30–38.

43. *Goldson L, Henrikson C O.* Root resorption during Begg treatment: a longitudinal roentgenologic study. *Am J Orthod* 1975; 68:55–66.

44. *Phillips J R.* Apical root resorption under orthodontic therapy. *Angle Orthod* 1955; 25:1–22.

45. *De Shields R W.* A study of root resorption in treated Class II, division I malocclusions. *Angle Orthod* 1969; 39:231–245.

46. *Massler M, Malone A J.* Root resorption in human permanent teeth. A roentgenographic study. *Am J Orthod* 1954; 40:619–633.

47. *Reitan K.* Biomechanical principles and reactions. In: Graber T M, Swain B F. *Current Orthodontic Concepts and Techniques.* Vol I. Philadelphia: W. B. Saunders Co; 1975; 111–229.

48. *Reitan K.* Initial tissue behavior during apical root resorption. *Angle Orthod* 1974; 44:68–82.

49. *Ten Hoeve A, Mulie R M.* The effect of antero-postero incisors repositioning on the palatal cortex, as studied with laminagraphy. *J Clin Orthod* 1976; 10:804–822.

50. *Andreasen J O.* Luxation of permanent teeth due to trauma. *Scand J Dent Res* 1970; 78:273–286.

51. *Bruszt P.* Secondary eruption of teeth intruded into the maxilla by a blow. *Oral Surg Oral Med Oral Pathol* 1958; 11:146–149.

52. *Cvek M.* Treatment of non-vital permanent incisors with calcium hydroxide. An effect on external root resorption in luxated teeth compared with effect of root filling with guttapercha, a follow-up. *Odontol Rev* 1973; 24:343–345.

53. *Ellis R G. The Classification and Treatment of Injuries to the Teeth of Children.* 2nd ed. Chicago: Year Book Medical Publ, Inc; 1948.

54. *Ravn J J.* Intrusion af permanente incisiver. *Tandlaegerbladet* 1975; 79:643–646.

55. *Skieller V.* The prognosis for young teeth loosened after mechanical injuries. *Acta Odontol Scan* 1960; 18:171–181.

56. *Snawder K.* Traumatic injuries to teeth of children. *J Prev Dent* 1976; 3:13–20.

57. *Turley P K, Joiner M W, Hellström S.* The effect of orthodontic extrusion on traumatically intruded teeth. *Am J Orthod* 1984; 85:47–56.

58. *Kristerson L.* Autotransplantation of human premolars: A clinical and radiographic study of 100 teeth. *Int J Oral Surg* 1985; 14:200–213.

59. *Lagerström L, Kristerson L.* Influence of orthodontic treatment on root development of autotransplanted premolars. *Am J Orthod* 1986; 89:146–150.

60. Malmgren O, Malmgren B, Frykholm A. Rapid orthodontic extrusion of crown root and cervical root fractured teeth. *Endod Dent Traumatol* 1991; 7:49–54.

Chapter 9

Autotransplantations and Orthodontic Treatment Planning

Jean-Paul Schatz / Jean-Pierre Joho

The early loss of permanent teeth, whether by trauma, decay, or congenital aplasia, has been usually corrected by prosthetic or orthodontic means. Though orthodontic treatment is always the best approach, in some cases the skeletal and dental relationship will contraindicate the use of space-closure mechanics to avoid a loss in the vertical dimension or the creation of a flat if not a dished-in facial profile (see chapter 3).

Because the prosthetic reconstructions are esthetically and functionally uncertain in the long-term, they should be discarded if possible in young patients. The use of autotransplantations, an ancient field of curiosity in dentistry, could be the ideal solution in specifically selected cases. The first scientific observations were made by Ambroise Paré in 1564 and by Hunter in 1776 in his *Natural History of Human Teeth,* describing procedures of worldwide interest. The 20th century marked the beginning of numerous basic experimental descriptions on immunology and histopathology of dental autotransplantations.

Principles

The treatment of choice for a total luxation in permanent dentition is the procedure of dental reimplantation, to avoid late prosthetic rehabilitation, which is sometimes complicated by dental migrations. A dental reimplantation follows rigorous schemes based on various experimental observations bearing analogies with the autotransplantation of teeth and dividing the responses to such a procedure in pulpal and periodontal reactions.

The trauma of a reimplantation can elicit severe pulpal damage, healed by various pulpodentinal reactions. Breivik[1] believes odontoblasts can survive perfectly to the reimplantation procedure, reparative dentin being already noticeable after 2 weeks in the apical third of the tooth. A wide-open root apex and a narrow pulp cavity seem to create favorable conditions for the healing processes: the pulp of immature teeth recovers vitality but revascularization very rarely takes place if root formation is completed. Kristerson and Andreasen[2] also point out the importance of pulp healing processes for root development. Microangiographic studies showed initial revascularization 4 days after reimplantation, extending to half of the pulp cavity after 10 days and to the whole pulp cavity after 30 days, mostly by migration of new blood vessels.[3, 4] Johnson and Burich[5] state in a recent study that negative photodensitometric recordings after 14 days indicate a definitive lack of revascularization.

Regeneration of nerve fibers is usually not observed before 1 month after a trauma, neither their number nor their diameter reaching normal levels. Vitality tests are therefore unreliable to disclose a possible pulp necrosis, discoloration of teeth and radiologically visible periapical rarefaction being more relevant. The pulp healing is obviously essential for the endodontic prognosis of reimplantation as well as for the periodontal healing, a major prognostic factor. With the help of the coagulum present after reimplantation, reorganized by young connective tissue, reattachment at the cementoenamel junction (CEJ) is possible after 1 week and healing of the periodontal breakdown is completed after 2 weeks. Numerous histologic studies describe the different modes of periodontal healing[6, 7]:

1. The root surface shows superficial resorption lacunae, transitory, self limited, and spontaneously repaired with new cementum. This so-called surface resorption, the most frequent response to localized injuries to the periodontal ligament, is histologically but not always radiographically seen. Its small size makes radiographic detection difficult. Those resorption cavities never reach the dentinal tubuli and allow a complete healing of the periodontium, without further evolution.

2. In cases with extensive damage to the periodontal ligament, whether mechanically or by desiccation, repopulation from adjacent bone marrow cells with osteo-

genic potential will lead to an ankylosis. Histologically, this fusion of alveolar bone and root surface can be demonstrated as soon as 2 weeks after reimplantation. This ankylosis, also called *replacement resorption,* can first be recognized radiographically at the apical third of the root 2 months after reimplantation. It can be progressive, gradually resorbing the entire root. In some instances, this process can be transient, when ankylosis is later resorbed by adjacent normal areas of the periodontium. Transient replacement resorption disappears within the first year and is followed by a recovery of the normal percussion sound. In contrast, an ankylosed tooth shows no mobility, infraocclusion, and a typical high percussion sound.

3. When resorptive processes are severe enough to connect dentinal tubuli and the periodontal tissues, a necrotic pulp can lead to rapidly progressive inflammatory resorption, an entire root being possibly resorbed within a few months. The inflammatory resorption cavities can be seen after 2 weeks at the apical third of the root, the tooth being clinically characterized by a strong mobility, extrusion, and sensitivity to percussion.

Autotransplantation and pulp vitality

The healing processes previously described don't strictly apply to the field of autotransplantation: the stage of root development is usually different, even if the reimplantation concerns a tooth with an open apex. Autotransplantation deals most often with a tooth bud before its eruption into the oral cavity, repositioned in an artificial socket somewhere else in the alveolar bone.

Revascularization progresses slowly, much slower than in the skin for instance. Large pulp areas survive through fluid metabolism and experience no vascularization during a few weeks. Castelli et al[8] observed permanent regressive pulp changes, though quote a fair revascularization in the apical third and perivascular bleeding leading to ischemia. This nutritional disturbance and the ensuing pathologies especially with a closed apex, may induce necrosis or inflammatory resorption.

In his histochemical study, Hasselgreen[9] confirms the work of Johnson by showing in the pulp cavity of mature transplanted teeth revascularization and pulp necrosis areas side by side. Skoglund, in studies already quoted, demonstrates a decrease of blood vessels between the 30th and the 180th day following transplantation, probably due to the initiation of pulp obliteration. In another study, Skoglund[10] tried to obtain a better revascularization of transplanted teeth by apicoectomy. Though his microangiographic results depicted the relative efficiency of this method, the vascular system is not as well and as rapidly restored than in teeth with an open apex. Many authors note that such a procedure does not enhance pulp cell survival, a lack of early anastomoses between pulp and periapical vessels being the main factor. The consecutive necrotic tissues are replaced by cells of the periapex and later by various hard tissue deposits. This pulp obliteration is histologically incomplete and may be followed by a secondary necrosis requiring endodontic treatment.

Breivik[1] recently described the processes leading to pulp obliteration, processes shown long ago by Sorg[11] and Øhman.[12] In the first 3 weeks following a reimplantation, destruction of the odontoblastic layer can be observed, some of it surviving with the help of the anaerobic pulpal metabolism, which maintains the continuity of the dentinal tubuli. The restoration of vascularization allows maturation of cells producing dentin: these new odontoblasts will be found in every part of the pulp chamber, with a strong predilection for the apical area in mature teeth with complete root formation. Apart from this reparative tissue, in various amount and quality, fibrous tissue is progressively replaced by calcified tissue, a protective mechanism against the periapical environment. Breivik points out the pulpal reaction to a trauma is always productive, the regenerating processes being more pronounced in young, immature teeth: deposition of secondary dentin is routine and reveals a strong pulpal healing potential.

Autotransplantation and periodontal healing

Northway[13] recently confirmed the overall belief in a physiologic incorporation of a transplant, where the prime prognostic factor is the integrity of the periodontium. According to Andreasen[7] and Andreasen and Kristerson,[14] the periodontal membrane of the cervical area is regenerated mainly by supracrestal connective tissue. He also confirmed the unique ability of periodontal membrane and follicular or gingival tissues to delay ankylosis and to induce cemental-type deposits. Various techniques have been used to control root resorption and the ankylosis phenomenon and to generate a normal periodontium. The use of tyrocalcitonine,[15] polylactic acid deposits, or elimination of antigenic components of the cemental matrix by hydrochlorate; none of these methods seem conclusive. Kahnberg[16] suggests the implantation of alveolar bone simultaneously with the transplantation in order to avoid root resorption, while Hansen and Fibaek[17] stress the importance of a tight gingival junction and the presence of alveolar bone, confirming the conclusions of Conklin.[18]

Cook[19] and Nasjleti[20] tried without success to promote periodontal healing by imbedding the transplant into the vestibular mucosa before autotransplantation. Andreasen,[14, 21] despite unsuccessful trials on histologic cultures of periodontal cells, also described transitory transplantations in the submucosa without preventing ankylosis and root resorption, nor allowing an adequate osseous neoformation along the periodontium. He considers these techniques as passive barriers between alveolar and radicular surfaces, possibly leading to premature exfoliation of the transplant.

In cases where healing progresses smoothly, osseous neoformation and gingival attachment are obvious, a normal periodontium being observed on the 30th day.[22] In young, immature teeth, a loose periodontal attachment should allow the healing processes by survival of a larger number of periodontal cells.

Therefore, most of the authors recommend the greatest care during the surgical procedure to avoid periodontal trauma and subsequent root resorption mechanisms. The cementum seems essential to the regeneration of a functional periodontium, and Dixon,[23] quoting Tonge,[24] attributes a prognostic factor to the distinctive characters of the cemental tissues in immature versus mature teeth.

Surgical procedure and technical considerations

Despite conflicting reports on prognostic factors of autotransplantations, many recent studies present obvious clinical success. In order to consider autotransplantation of teeth as part of orthodontic treatment planning, a proper surgical technique seems of utmost importance.[25]

Though the surgical procedure may denote some minor modifications, the operation, performed under local anesthesia, follows the same basic steps:
1. Mobilization of the transplant
2. Preparation of the receiver site
3. Removal and transfer of the donor tooth
4. Suturing of the mucoperiosteal flap
5. Fixation of the transplant (see chapter 4 for basic surgical principles)

In certain cases, local conditions may limit the preparation of an ideal artificial socket, thus requiring the positioning of the transplant in slight rotation later corrected by orthodontic means. Moreover, the marked involution of the alveolar bone will lead to an extensive osseous cortical breakdown, a situation often seen in transplantation of impacted canines. Because divergent opinions are expressed by periodontists in studies dealing with the ability of the periodontium to restore normal periodontal conditions,[26, 27] it seems advisable to respect as much as possible the alveolar bone level during that surgical step.

The survival of the periodontal ligament being critical, the extraction of the transplant must be done cautiously, with care being taken to avoid the use of surgical tools or techniques detrimental to the CEJ or to the periodontal healing.

With no satisfactory method described in the literature to prevent resorption processes, we only recommend postoperative prophylactic antibiotherapy, which, associated with maintenance of a perfect hygiene, will reduce the risk of a pulp necrosis and a possible inflammatory resorption.

The period of fixation, by various means but preferably with fixed orthodontic appliances, must be reduced to achieve the restoration of the periodontal support without root resorptions.[28, 29]

Indications

In young patients where prosthetic reconstruction should be postponed, autotransplantations become in selected cases an excellent solution to orthodontic problems complicated by missing teeth. There are numerous clinical studies and case reports dealing with autotransplantations, showing different types of transplanted teeth applied to a specific clinical situation and covering a large field of indications.

Since the decisive work of Apfel[30, 31] reporting transplantations of third molar buds into extraction sites of first permanent molars, Slagsvold and Bjercke,[32, 33] and later Nordenram,[34, 35] started premolar transplantations in orthodontic problem cases. Though each kind of tooth can be a transplant adapted to a given situation, the morphology of premolars is such that the ideal transplants for these teeth are other premolars. Though essentially used in clinical disharmonies where crowding is combined with congenitally missing premolars, those tooth buds can, according to various authors, replace canines or incisors. Slagsvold[36] presented cases where congenitally missing maxillary lateral incisors were replaced by mandibular incisors, a similar situation being possible when maxillary incisors are lost as a result of trauma. Because the prognoses are always uncertain and because of the prosthetic complications, autotransplantations should be only undertaken in selected orthodontic cases.

According to Slagsvold,[33] premolar root formation should have started (one fourth to one third complete) in order to increase success rates. Hence, the ideal stage seems to be when root formation is half completed, still allowing a sufficient root growth. Slagsvold sees third molar buds as acceptable transplants for lost first molars or for premolars, while Northway[13] considers the fully formed wisdom teeth as ideal transplants because a late formation allows their use in young adults. Numerous descriptions are shown in the literature, demonstrating a wide variety of clinical indications.

Supernumerary teeth (mesiodens, etc) can also be transplanted to replace missing teeth,[37] though some anatomic considerations such as root underdevelopment or malformation may often restrict their use.

Several reports have been made on surgical repositioning of canines since Widman[38] presented cases of autotransplanted impacted canines. Various problems related to the age of the patient, the stage of root formation at the time of autotransplantation, and the localization of the impacted canine may directly affect the prognosis. However, this procedure is still a

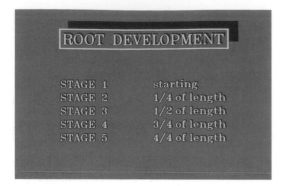

Fig. 9-1

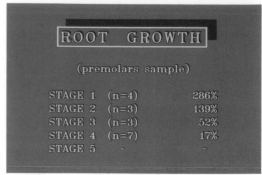

Fig. 9-2

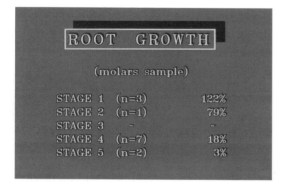

Fig. 9-3

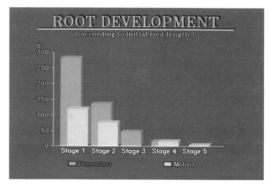

Fig. 9-4

major therapeutic tool in desperate cases of impactions or failure of orthodontic repositioning.

Conclusions

The results of our own radiologic survey confirmed the conclusions of the various authors quoted in this chapter, in regard to the importance of proper timing to ensure periodontal and pulpal healing and final root growth. Pulpal healing is related, as mentioned in most of the studies, to the stage of root edification (Fig. 9-1), and our

results match those of Kristerson[2] or Schwartz[25]: every transplanted tooth but two maintained vitality and underwent partial or total pulpal obliteration. As in Kristerson's and Schwartz's studies, this phenomenon was observed primarily in young, immature teeth, because of a wide apical foramen and an easier revascularization pathway.

Our transplants all demonstrated continuous root growth (Figs. 9-2 to 9-4), although slightly less than in Kristerson's sample, but in a same range as noted by Slagsvold and Bjercke.[33] According to these researchers, premolar transplantations performed at any stage before com-

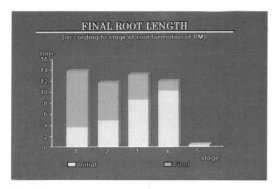

Fig. 9-5

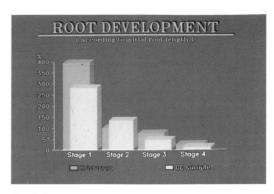

Fig. 9-6

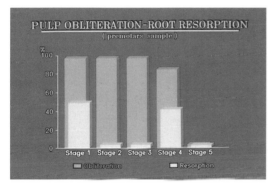

Fig. 9-7

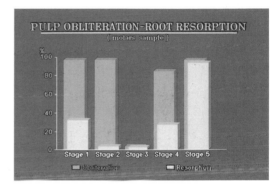

Fig. 9-8

plete root formation allow continued root development. Final root length will only be 10 % shorter when compared to contralateral teeth (Fig. 9-5). Those findings have been supported by Kristerson[2] in a long-term study of 100 autotransplanted premolars, confirming good prognoses when performed at one half to three fourths of root length. Some genetic factors seem to control the process of root growth, and we concur with Slagsvold and Bjercke[32, 33] that a tooth transplant can reach its final root length when the surgical procedure is performed under optimal conditions.

Our sample showed continuous root growth, with persistence of vitality, though

root formation appeared slightly reduced compared to Kristerson's findings (Fig. 9-6): the results lead us to consider the transplantation of premolars at stages 2 and 3, and the transplantation of molars at stage 4, a compromise between maximal root growth after transplantation and optimal periodontal healing.

Although our inflammatory resorption rate is extremely low, the percentage of ankylosis is higher than Kristerson's or Slagsvold's data, but compare favorably to Schwartz's work (Figs. 9-7 and 9-8).

The autotransplantations of canines and of teeth with complete root edification usually necessitate endodontic root canal

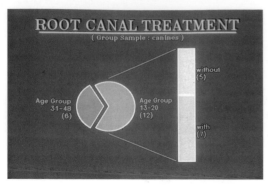

Fig. 9-9

treatment to avoid pulpal necrosis and inflammatory resorption processes (Fig. 9-9). The surgical procedure often being complicated in those cases, the periodontal support, as evaluated by vertical bone resorption and gingival height, is compromised. It seems therefore essential to increase the success rate by carefully planning autotransplantation in orthodontic cases as early as possible, respecting the already mentioned factors of prognostic value. Because of careful radiologic screening and routine endodontic treatments, we did not observe inflammatory resorption and saw a replacement resorption rate similar to Altonen[39] when dealing with canine autotransplantations.

Autotransplantations can be considered a major tool in orthodontic armamentarium, reducing the severity of some orthodontic cases while respecting other therapeutic means without compromising the dental status in case of failure.

Apart from a perfect understanding of the treatment's considerations and prognosis by patient and family, the only prerequisite is the maintenance of rigorous buccal hygiene on a long-term basis. Transplantations of teeth can then represent a reasonable therapy solving, as shown in the following case reports, the problems raised by aplasias or traumatic loss of teeth in specific clinical situations.

Case reports

Case 1 (Figs. 9-10a to q)

At the initial consultation, this 11½-year-old girl had a skeletal and dental Class I relationship and aplasia of teeth (Figs. 9-10a to e). Treatment planning aimed at keeping the dental Class I relationship by closing the spaces of missing 31–41 with a full fixed-appliance therapy, together with the transplantation of 24 in situ 35 and the prosthetic reconstruction of missing 45. Figures 9-10f to j show the final results immediately posttransplantation and at the end of the orthodontic treatment. Figures 9-10k to q present the long-term clinical and radiological results.

Case 2 (Figs. 9-11a to o)

This 14½-year-old boy had an impacted lower canine with a dental and skeletal Class I relationship (Figs. 9-11a to e). Because the orthodontic disimpaction bore some risks for the integrity of the mandibular incisors, it was decided to open the space for the transplantation of 43 (Figs. 9-11f to j).

The long-term clinical and radiologic results are presented in Figs. 9-11k to o.

Figs. 9-10a and b   Frontal view and initial radiological screening

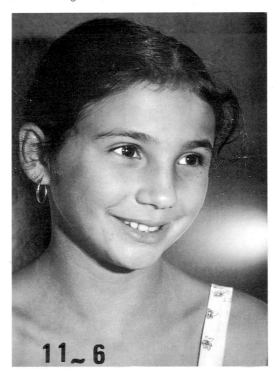

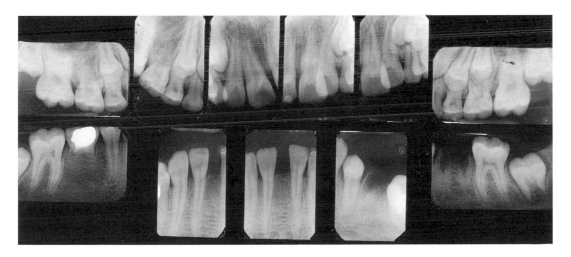

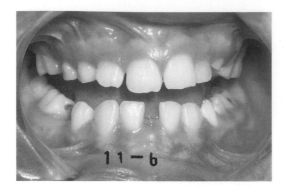

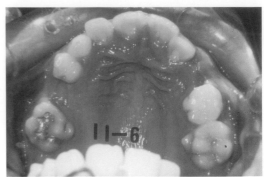

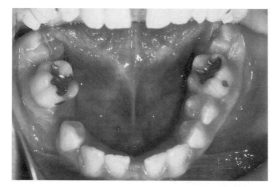

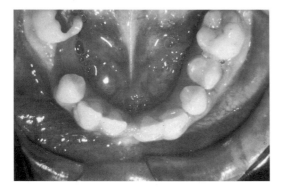

Figs. 9-10c to e   Initial intraoral views.

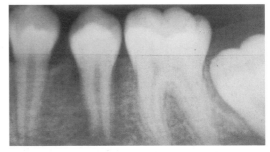

Figs. 9-10f and g   Clinical and radiological views posttransplantation.

Figs. 9-10h to j   Intraoral views at the end of the orthodontic treatment. Bilateral Class I relationship before prosthetic rehabilitation.

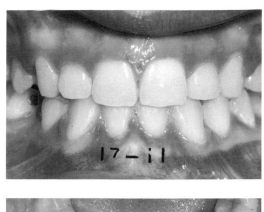

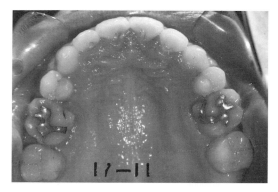

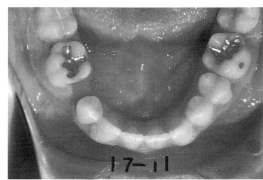

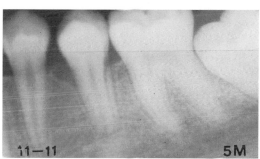

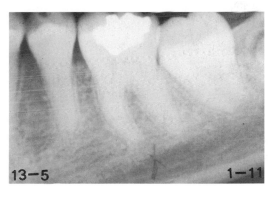

Figs. 9-10k to m   Radiological views at 5 months; 1 year, 11 months; and 6 years, 5 months after transplantation.

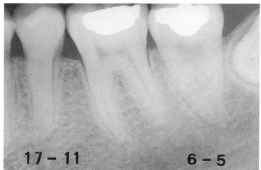

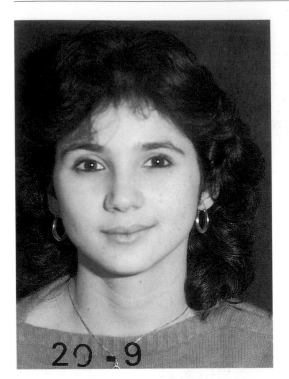

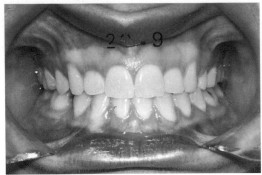

Figs. 9-10n to q   Clinical and radiological controls at the 9 year, 3 month postoperative followup.

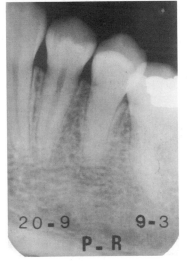

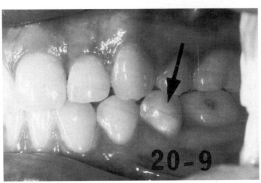

Figs. 9-11a and b   Frontal view and initial orthopan-tomograph.

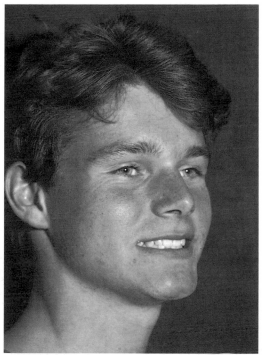

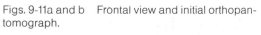

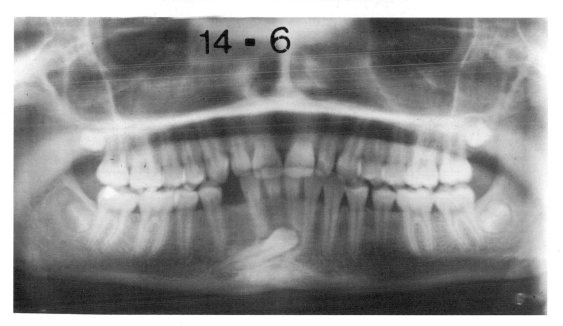

Figs. 9-11c to e   Initial intraoral views.

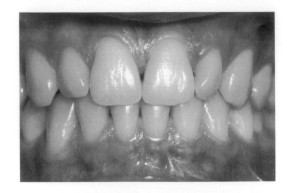

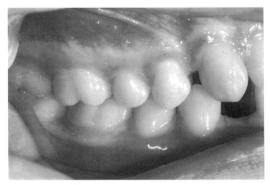

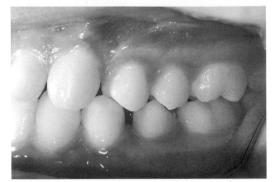

Figs. 9-11f to h   Clinical views after orthodontic space opening.

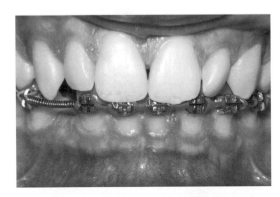

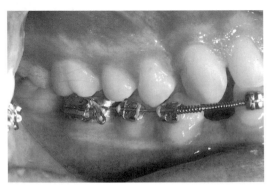

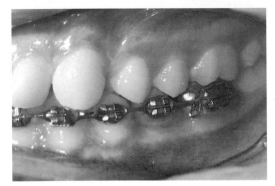

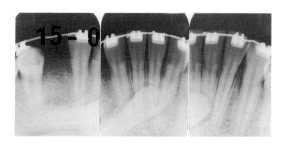

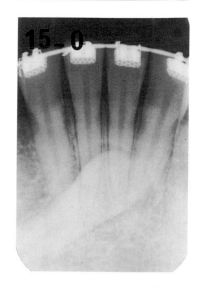

Figs. 9-11i and j   Radiological views before transplantation.

Figs. 9-11k to m   Intraoral views 2 years after transplantation.

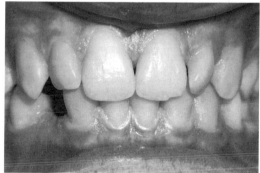

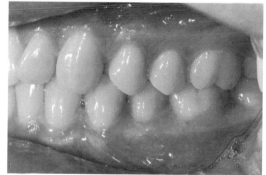

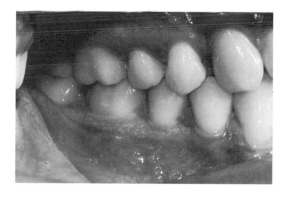

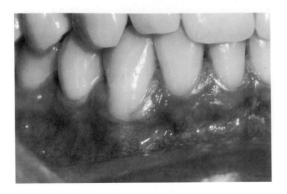
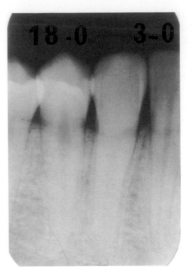

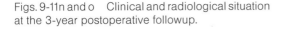

Figs. 9-11n and o   Clinical and radiological situation at the 3-year postoperative followup.

References

1. *Breivik M.* Human odontoblast response to tooth replantation. *Eur J Orthod* 1981; 3:95–108.
2. *Kristerson L.* Autotransplantation of human premolars. A clinical and radiographic study of 100 teeth. *Int J Oral Surg* 1985; 14:200–213.
3. *Skoglund A.* Pulp reactions in reimplanted and autotransplanted teeth of dogs. Malmö, Sweden: University of Malmö; 1980. Thesis.
4. *Skoglund A, Tronstad L, Wallenius K.* A microangiographic study of vascular changes in replanted and autotransplanted teeth of young dogs. *Oral Surg Oral Med Oral Pathol* 1978; 45:17–27.
5. *Johnson D S, Burich R L.* Revascularization of reimplanted teeth in dogs. *J Dent Res* 1979; 58:671.
6. *Andreasen J O.* Traumatic Injuries of the Teeth. 2nd ed. Copenhagen: Munksgaard; 1981a.
7. *Andreasen J O.* Periodontal healing after replantation and autotransplantation of permanent incisors. *Int J Oral Surg* 1981b; 10:54–61.
8. *Castelli WA, Nasjleti CE, Caffesse RG, Dias-Perez R.* Vascular response of the periodontal membrane after replantation of teeth. *Oral Surg Oral Med Oral Pathol* 1980; 50:390–397.
9. *Hasselgren G, Larsson Å, Rundquist L.* Pulpal status after autogenous transplantation of fully developed maxillary canines. *Oral Surg Oral Med Oral Pathol* 1977; 44:106–112.
10. *Skoglund A.* Vascular changes in replanted and autotransplanted apicoectomized mature teeth of dogs. *Int J Oral Surg* 1981; 10:100–110.
11. *Sorg W R.* Nerve regeneration in replanted hamster teeth. *J Dent Res* 1960; 39:1222–1231.
12. *Øhman A.* Healing and Sensitivity to Pain in Young Replanted Human Teeth. *An Experimental, Clinical and Histological Study.* Gothenburg, Sweden: University of Gothenburg; 1965. Thesis.
13. *Northway W M, Konigsberg S.* Autogenetic tooth transplantation. The "state of the art." *Am J Orthod* 1980; 77:146–162.
14. *Andreasen J O, Kristeron L.* Evaluation of different types of autotransplanted connective tissues as potential periodontal ligament substitutes. *Int J Oral Surg* 1981; 10:189–201.
15. *Andreasen J O, Schwartz O, Andreasen F M.* The effect of apicoectomy before replantation and pulpal healing in monkeys. *Int J Oral Surg* 1985; 14:176–183.
16. *Kahnberg KE, Warfvinge J, Birgersson B.* Intraalveolar transplantation. The use of autologous bone transplants in the periapical region. *Int J Oral Maxillofac Surg* 1987; 16:577–585.
17. *Hansen J, Fibaek B.* Clinical experience of auto- and allotransplantation of teeth. *Int Dent J* 1972; 22:270–285.
18. *Conklin W W.* Long-term follow-up and evaluation of transplantation of fully developed teeth. *Oral Surg Oral Med Oral Pathol* 1978; 46:477–485.

19. *Cook R M.* The current status of autogenous transplantation as applied to the maxillary canine. *Int Dent J* 1972; 22:286–300.

20. *Nasjleti C E, Caffesse R G, Castelli W A.* Replantation of mature teeth without endodontics in monkeys. *J Dent Res* 1978; 57:650–658.

21. *Andreasen J O.* The effect of extraalveolar period and storage media upon periodontal and pulpal healing after replantation of mature permanent incisors in monkeys. *Int J Oral Surg* 1981; 10:43–53.

22. *Löe H, Waerhaug J.* Experimental replantation ot teeth in dogs and monkeys. *Arch Oral Biol* 1961; 3:176–184.

23. *Dixon D A.* Autogenous transplantation of tooth germs into the upper incisor region. *Br Dent J* 1971; 131:260–265.

24. *Tonge C H.* Advances in dental embryology. *Int Dent J* 1966; 16:328.

25. *Schwartz O, Bergmann P, Klausen B.* Autotransplantation of human teeth. A life table analysis of prognostic factors. *Int J Oral Surg* 1985a; 14:245–258.

26. *Andreasen J O.* Interrelation between alveolar bone and periodontal ligament repair after replantation of mature permanent incisors in monkeys. *J Period Res* 1981; 16:228–235.

27. *Lindhe J, Nyman S, Karring T.* Connective tissue reattachment as related to presence or absence of alveolar bone. *J Clin Periodontol* 1984; 11:33–40.

28. *Andersson L, Lindskog S, Blomlöf L, et al:* Effect of masticatory stimulation on dentoalveolar ankylosis after experimental tooth replantation. *Endod Dent Traumatol* 1985; 1:13–16.

29. *Andreasen J O.* The effect of splinting upon periodontal healing after replantation of permanent incisors in monkeys. *Acta Odont Scand* 1975; 33:313–323.

30. *Apfel H.* Preliminary work in transplanting the third molar to the first molar position. *J Am Dent Assoc* 1954; 48:143–150.

31. *Apfel H.* Autoplasty of enucleated prefunctional third molars. *J Oral Surg* 1950; 8:289–296.

32. *Slagsvold O, Bjercke B.* Indications for autotransplantation in cases of missing premolars. *Am J Orthod* 1978a; 74:241–257.

33. *Slagsvold O, Bjercke B.* Autotransplantation of premolars with partly formed roots. *Am J Orthod* 1974; 66:355–366.

34. *Nordenram A.* Autotransplantation of teeth. A clinical and experimental investigation. *Acta Odont Scand* 1963; 22(suppl):33.

35. *Nordenram A.* Autotransplantation of teeth. *Br J Oral Surg* 1969; 7:188–195.

36. *Slagsvold O, Bjercke B.* Applicability of autotransplantation in cases of missing upper anterior teeth. *Am J Orthod* 1978b; 74:410–421.

37. *Taylor G S.* Autotransplant replacement of a geminated incisor by a supplemental incisor. *Br J Orthod* 1979; 6:195–198.

38. *Widman L.* Om transplantation av retinerade hörntänder. *Svensk Tandläkare Tidskrift* 1915; 8:289–296.

39. *Altonen M, Haavikko K, Malmström M.* Evaluation of autotransplantations of completely developed maxillary canines. Int J Oral Surg 1978; 7:434–441.

Index

183